The Biological Affinities of the Eastern Mediterranean in the Chalcolithic and Bronze Age

The Biological Affinities of the Eastern Mediterranean in the Chalcolithic and Bronze Age

A Regional Dental Non-metric Approach

Zissis Parras

BAR International Series 1305
2004

Published in 2016 by
BAR Publishing, Oxford

BAR International Series 1305

The Biological Affinities of the Eastern Mediterranean in the Chalcolithic and Bronze Age

ISBN 978 1 84171 382 3

© Z Parras and the Publisher 2004

The author's moral rights under the 1988 UK Copyright,
Designs and Patents Act are hereby expressly asserted.

All rights reserved. No part of this work may be copied, reproduced, stored,
sold, distributed, scanned, saved in any form of digital format or transmitted
in any form digitally, without the written permission of the Publisher.

BAR Publishing is the trading name of British Archaeological Reports (Oxford) Ltd.
British Archaeological Reports was first incorporated in 1974 to publish the BAR
Series, International and British. In 1992 Hadrian Books Ltd became part of the BAR
group. This volume was originally published by John and Erica Hedges Ltd. in
conjunction with British Archaeological Reports (Oxford) Ltd / Hadrian Books Ltd,
the Series principal publisher, in 2004. This present volume is published by BAR
Publishing, 2016.

Printed in England

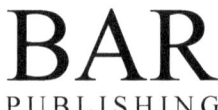

BAR titles are available from:

        BAR Publishing
        122 Banbury Rd, Oxford, OX2 7BP, UK
EMAIL   info@barpublishing.com
PHONE +44 (0)1865 310431
  FAX   +44 (0)1865 316916
        www.barpublishing.com

Dedicated to the memory of Anna Diamantakos

1965-2001

ABSTRACT

This study investigated biological population affinities amongst Eastern Mediterranean Chalcolithic and Bronze Age human skeletal samples. Seven hundred and eighty-six human remains from eight different sites in Cyprus, Greece and Syria were studied. The sites range in age from the Cypriot Chalcolithic (Souskiou-Vathyrkakas, Lemba-Lakkous and Kissonerga-Mosphilia) to Cypriot Late Bronze Age (Enkomi and Ayios Iakovos), Syrian Early Bronze (Jerablus-Tahtani) and Greek Middle Bronze Ages (Lerna and Asine). Age, sex and non-metric traits from the dentition, crania and post-crania were recorded. Using the non-metric dental data the biological affinities of these sites were determined. Two statistics were utilised with the non-metric traits to determine biological affinities, the Mean Measure of Divergence (MMD) and the Coefficient of θ ($D.\theta$). The comparisons between the sites from southwest Cyprus show all three sites, which are in close spatial proximity, to be statistically biologically similar. Also they appeared to show some relation to the Syrian Early Bronze age site of Jerablus-Tahtani. These findings are in contrast to the different material cultures of these two regions, which may suggest the biological relation, may be based on the ancestral contact between Cyprus and the mainland. The Cypriot Late Bronze sites show a mixed relation with the Chalcolithic samples with some relations with the Middle Bronze Age Greek samples and Syria. Where geographical distance is usually a factor in these types of comparisons, this study suggests time may also be a factor.

ACKNOWLEDGEMENTS

I would like to begin by saying that my Ph.D. experience has been an amazing journey. Over 700 human remains were studied from 3 countries, with trips to Scotland, Greece, Cyprus and Sweden for data collection. This study represents the successful combination of physical anthropology with archaeology to produce a unique union of the two.

I would first like to extend my warmest gratitude to my two supervisors Andrew Chamberlain and Paul Halstead. Their guidance and encouragement over these past few years have been invaluable. Also the administration at the Department of Archaeology (and Prehistory) at the University of Sheffield has been very kind and accommodating. I am especially thankful to Kathryn Goldsack (Graduate School) for her helpful and positive attitude. Thanks very much, you made the whole PhD process 10 times easier. I would also like to extend thanks to Prof. Barbara S. Ottaway the former head of the Research School and Prof. Paul Buckland the current head. Prof. Keith Branigan and Dr. Peter Day with their help with getting access to human remains for Greece. Dr. Martin Evison, Dept of Forensic Pathology (University of Sheffield), whose correspondence was very helpful in formulating the method of this PhD. Dr Terence Brown from the University of Manchester (Biomolecular Sciences – UMIST) for his helpful correspondence on the possibility of extracting ancient DNA from human bones and teeth.

I would also like to thank some friends from the University of Sheffield who were very helpful with this study. Dr. Eva Panagiotakopulu was always helpful and supportive. Dr. Sevi Triantaphyllou assisted me with our discussions about how to conduct the data collection of the human remains. Dr. Yiannis Papadatos was most helpful with the many discussions on possible collections of human remains from Greece. Dr. Andy Tyrrell was very helpful in the statistical approach to this study. Finally Costa Eliopoulos whose friendship and support throughout the many years in England, Greece and Canada were invaluable.

I would also like to thank Prof. Eddy J. Peltenburg of the University of Edinburgh who allowed me access to the samples from Cyprus of Lemba-Lakkous and Kissonerga-Mosphilia and Jerablus-Tahtani from Syria. His support and comments on my thesis and his help in granting me access to the human remains from Souskiou-Vathyrkakas (Cyprus) are appreciated, as well as allowing me to stay at the Lemba Archaeological Research Centre on two trips to Cyprus. Also am grateful for the use of the facilities at the Archaeology department at the University of Edinburgh. I would also like to thank Drs. Dorothy Lunt and Marie Watt of The University of Glasgow Dental School. Dr. Lunt for her friendly correspondence, continuous help and advice, and for allowing me access to The University of Glasgow Dental School and its facilities to study the remains from Jerablus-Tahtani and Souskiou-Vathyrkakas.

Thanks to the British Council for Research in the Levant who gave me my only grant which I used for one trip to Cyprus. My two trips to Cyprus were very productive at the Lemba Archaeological Research Centre. I would also like to extend a very special thanks to Dr. Paul Croft for his tremendous help and friendliness. He kindly drove me around when I didn't have use of a car and was kind enough to share some of his time for our discussions of Cypriot archaeology. I would also wish to thank Dr. Vasiliki Kassianidou of the Archaeological Research Unit, University of Cyprus for putting me in touch with Paul Croft, Dr. Sophocles Hadjisavvas Director Department of Antiquities in Cyprus, his correspondence and generosity in allowing me access to the remains of Lemba and Mosphilia at the Paphos Museum. Also special thanks to the Director and staff from the Paphos Museum for their kindness and helpful nature. They made working there a very pleasant affair. Also thanks to Eleni Louka and Elena Prokopiou from the Archaeological Museum at Lemesos. Thanks to Eleni for taking me to Larnaka Museum to meet the people there.

I also wish to thank Dr. Martha H. Wiencke, Director of the Lerna Publications Project who allowed me access to the human remains from Lerna and helped with my application to the Ephoria. Thanks to the Nauplion Ephoria and Dr. Elisabet Spathari for allowing me access to the human remains from Lerna, which are being housed at the museum of Argos. Thanks to the staff at the Museum of Argos for their prompt and friendly assistance. I would also wish to thank the manager and staff at the Hotel Mycenan in Argos, where I stayed while I studied the collection from Lerna at the museum. Thanks for our long conversations about archaeology and history.

My trip to Sweden was very enjoyable and productive, with special thanks to Anne Ingvarsson-Sundström of Uppsala University and her husband Andres. Anne was generous enough to allow me access to some of her research on the human remains from Asine and she did all of the work of going through Prof. Persson's notebook and others site books (in Swedish) to determine provenience and other details of the original excavation. Thanks to Anne's friend Lena Johansson in Uppsala who let me stay at her house for the week I was there. I appreciated the use of the facilities at Uppsala University and the Library. It was a pleasure to meet with Prof. Gullög C. Nordquist also at Uppsala University. I would also like to thank Marie-Louise Windbladh curator of the Museum of Mediterranean and Near Eastern Antiquities,

Medelhavsmuseet, Stockholm and her assistant Ole Sylvean who allowed me access to the human remains from Enkomi and Ayios Iakovos (Cyprus) from the Swedish Expedition in the 1920's. I would like to thank the photographer who was kind enough to supply me with photographs of some of the human remains. I appreciate all the help and kindness from Dr. Karin Niklasson Hägg and Prof. Robin Hägg of the University of Göteborg during my time spent in Göteborg studying the human remains from Enkomi and Ayios Iakovos. Also thanks to Professor Paul Åstrom for allowing me to purchase some volumes from the Studies in Mediterranean Archaeology series at a reduced rate.

Some others must also be thanked, Prof. Dave Smith, Prof. Jerry Melbye and Prof. B.A. Sigmon from the University of Toronto at Mississauga (Anthropology Department) whose support and encouragement was greatly appreciated. Also Dr. Todd Morris, Department of Biology (University of Toronto Department of Biology) who help with statistics was also appreciated. Dr. Wim van Neer of The Royal Museum of Central Africa in Tervuren (Belgium) whose letter of reference helped me get accepted to the University of Sheffield. I am also grateful for the University of Toronto Library system for help with my research. I would also like to thank The Metropolitan Toronto Reference Library, Mississauga Library, Working Ventures Inc. and Tim Horton's Inc. I would also like to extend a special thanks to Dr. David Reese of the Field Museum of Natural History, Chicago Illinois. I have known Dr, Reese since 1995, but we have never met in person. He has regularly sent me relevant articles regarding my thesis topic and given me much information regarding skeletal collections and excavations in the Eastern Mediterranean. Special thanks also goes out to the many people on the archaeology news group Aegeanet, their discussions and information about where to look for human remains and their kind comments on my web site (Physical Anthropology of the Eastern Mediterranean during the Bronze Age). Also thanks to the hundred or so people that I wrote, emailed and faxed, who assisted in small but meaningful ways.

I am grateful to both of my examiners Drs. Glynis Jones and Dr. John E. Robb who both gave me such positive and constructive feedback during my defense. They made the defense one of the most positive experiences in my life. Also their suggestions regarding the corrections for my thesis really added in the overall cohesiveness of the work.

Overall I would like to extend gratitude to my parents and to my entire family whose total and unwavering support and commitment to my studies has been invaluable. Finally the warmest thanks to my dearest wife Aida, whose support cannot be explained in words and has been with me since the beginning of my studies who never lost sight of the end even when I did.

LIST OF CONTENTS

DEDICATION	i
ABSTRACT	iii
ACKNOWLEDGEMENTS	iv
LIST OF CONTENTS	vii
LIST OF TABLES	xii
LIST OF FIGURES	xiii
ABBREVIATION	xiii
CHAPTER 1: INTRODUCTION	1
1.1 Principal Aims	1
1.2 Archaeological Questions	2
1.3 Method	2
CHAPTER 2: TIME PERIOD, REGION AND SKELETAL SAMPLES	3
2.1 Introduction	3
2.2 Cyprus:	3
2.2.1 Souskiou	3
2.2.1.1 Location	3
2.2.1.2 Setting	4
2.2.1.3 History	4
2.2.1.4 Time Period	4
2.2.1.5 Type of Site	4
2.2.1.6 Location, type and number of tombs	4
2.2.1.7 Grave Goods	5
2.2.2 Lemba-Lakkous	5
2.2.2.1 Location	5
2.2.2.2 Setting	5
2.2.2.3 History	5
2.2.2.4 Time Period	5
2.2.2.5 Type of Site	6
2.2.2.6 Location, type and number of tombs	6
2.2.2.7 Grave Goods	6
2.2.3 Kissonerga-Mosphilia	6
2.2.3.1 Location	6
2.2.3.2 Setting	7
2.2.3.3 History	7
2.2.3.4 Time Period	7
2.2.3.5 Type of Site	7
2.2.3.6 Location, type and number of tombs	7
2.2.3.7 Grave Goods	8
2.2.4 Ayios Iakovos	8
2.2.4.1 Location	8
2.2.4.2 Setting	8
2.2.4.3 History	8
2.2.4.4 Time Period	8
2.2.4.5 Type of Site	8
2.2.4.6 Location, type and number of tombs	8
2.2.4.7 Grave Goods	9
2.2.5 Enkomi	9
2.2.5.1 Location	9
2.2.5.2 Setting	9
2.2.5.3 History	9
2.2.5.4 Time Period	9
2.2.5.5 Type of Site	9
2.2.5.6 Location, type and number of tombs	9

2.2.5.7 Grave Goods	9
2.2.6 Summary	9
2.2.6.1 Chalcolithic Cyprus	9
2.2.6.2 Late Bronze Age	10
2.3 Greece:	10
2.3.1 Asine	10
2.3.1.1 Location	10
2.3.1.2 Setting	10
2.3.1.3 History	10
2.3.1.4 Time Period	10
2.3.1.5 Type of Site	10
2.3.1.6 Location, type and number of tombs	11
2.3.1.7 Grave Goods	11
2.3.2 Lerna	11
2.3.2.1 Location	11
2.3.2.2 Setting	11
2.3.2.3 History	11
2.3.2.4 Time Period	11
2.3.2.5 Type of Site	12
2.3.2.6 Location, type and number of tombs	12
2.3.2.7 Grave Goods	12
2.3.3 Summary	12
2.4 Syria:	12
2.4.1 Jerablus-Tahtani	13
2.4.1.1 Location	13
2.4.1.2 Setting	13
2.4.1.3 History	13
2.4.1.4 Time Period	13
2.4.1.5 Type of Site	13
2.4.1.6 Location, type and number of tombs	13
2.4.1.7 Grave Goods	14
2.4.2 Summary	14
CHAPTER 3: ANTHROPOLOGICAL METHODS	**15**
3.1. Introduction	15
3.2. State of Preservation	15
3.3. Minimum Number of Individuals (MNI)	15
3.4. Age Estimation	16
3.4.1. Age Estimation Methods	16
3.4.2. Age Groups	16
3.5. Sex Determination	17
3.6. Demography	17
3.7. Stature	18
3.8. Non-Metric Traits	18
3.8.1. Introduction	18
3.8.2. Side Considerations	18
3.8.3. Sex Considerations	19
3.8.4. Age Differences	19
3.8.5. Dental Non-Metric Traits	19
3.8.6. Cranial Non-Metric Traits	20
3.8.7. Post-cranial Non-Metric Traits	21
3.8.8. Problems with Trait collection	21
3.9. Data from publications	21
3.10 Other sources of genetic data	21
3.11 Cranial Metrics	22
CHAPTER 4: DEMOGRAPHY	**23**
4.1. Introduction	23

4.2. South-west Cyprus	23
4.2.1 Souskiou	23
4.2.2 Lemba-Lakkous	23
4.2.3 Kissonerga-Mosphilia	24
4.2.4 South West Cyprus Demography	24
4.2.5 Adult Mortality	25
4.2.6 Kolmogorov-Smirnov Test	26
4.2.7 Other Cypriot Sites	27
4.2.8 Kolmogorov-Smirnov Test	28
4.2.9 Summary	30
4.3 Regional Comparison	30
4.3.1 Jerablus-Tahtani	30
4.3.2 Jerablus-Tahtani Mortality	30
4.3.3 Anatolia	30
4.3.4 Adult Mortality for Syria and Anatolia	32
4.3.5 Kolmogorov-Smirnov Test	32
4.3.6 Summary	32
4.4 Aegean Sites	33
4.4.1 Asine	33
4.4.2 Lerna	33
4.4.3 Ayios Kosmas	33
4.4.4 Kephala	33
4.4.5 Greek Mortality	33
4.4.6 Adult Mortality for Greece	34
4.4.7 Kolmogorov-Smirnov Test	35
4.4.8 Summary	36
4.5 Late Bronze Age North East Cyprus	36
4.5.1 Ayios Iakovos	36
4.5.2 Enkomi	36
4.5.3 Mortality	36
4.5.4 Adult Mortality	37
4.5.5 Kolmogorov-Smirnov Test	37
4.5.6 Summary	38
4.6 Chapter Summary	38
4.6.1 Southwest Cyprus	38
4.6.2 Northeast Cyprus	38
4.6.3 Greece	39
4.6.4 Syria	39
CHAPTER 5: STATURE AND NON-METRICS	**40**
5.1 Stature	40
5.1.1 Introduction	40
5.1.2 Male Stature	40
5.1.3 Female Stature	40
5.1.4 Combined Male and Female Stature	42
5.1.5 Regional Stature Comparison	42
5.1.6 Summary	43
5.2 Cranial and Post-Cranial Non-Metric Traits	44
5.2.1 Introduction	44
5.2.2 Cranial Non-Metrics	44
5.2.3 Other samples around the Eastern Mediterranean	45
5.2.4 Summary	46
5.3 Post-Cranial Non-Metric Traits	46
5.3.1 Introduction	46
5.3.2 Comparison	46
5.4 Summary	47

CHAPTER 6: BIO-DISTANCE — 48
6.1. Introduction — 48
    6.1.1 Mean Measure of Divergence — 48
    6.1.2 Coefficient of "θ" — 49
6.2 $D.\theta$ Analysis — 49
    6.2.1 Summary — 52
6.3 Mean Measure of Divergence Analysis — 52
    6.3.1 Summary — 53
6.4 Discussion of the $D.\theta$ and the MMD — 55
6.5 Comparison with other sites — 56
    6.5.1 The $D.\theta$ Comparison with other sites — 56
    6.5.2 The MMD Comparison with other sites — 58
    6.5.3 Summary of the $D.\theta$ and the MMD Regional comparison — 60

CHAPTER 7: DISCUSSION — 61
7.1. Introduction — 61
    7.2.1. Chalcolithic Cyprus — 61
    7.2.2 Anthropological and DNA Evidence — 62
    7.2.3. Summary — 64
7.3. The Archaeological Evidence — 64
    7.3.1. Earliest Connections with the Mainland — 64
        7.3.1.1. Subsistence Pattern — 65
        7.3.1.2. Artefacts — 65
        7.3.1.3. Burials — 65
        7.3.1.4. Houses and Architecture — 66
    7.3.2. Evidence of Cypriot artefacts on the mainland — 66
    7.3.3. Summary — 66
7.4. Late Neolithic Sotira and Chalcolithic Erimi cultures — 67
    7.4.1. End of the Khirokitia Culture — 67
    7.4.2. Sotira Culture — 67
    7.4.3. Erimi Culture — 67
    7.4.4. Evidence for contact with the mainland — 68
    7.4.5. End of the Chalcolithic — 68
    7.4.6. Summary — 68
7.5. Middle Bronze Greece and Late Bronze Age Cyprus — 69
    7.5.1. Dental Non-Metric Evidence — 69
    7.5.2. Contacts with the Aegean during the Bronze Age — 70
    7.5.3. Contacts with the Aegean during the Late Bronze Age — 70
    7.5.4. Contacts with the Mainland in the Late Bronze Age — 71
7.6. Artificial Cranial Deformation — 71
    7.6.1. Summary — 72

CHAPTER 8: CONCLUSION — 73
8.1 Recommendations for Future Research — 74
8.2 Conclusions from using this kind of data — 74

REFERENCES — 75

APPENDIX
1. Chronology Table of all regions — 88
2. Chronology of Cyprus — 89
3. Non-metric Cranial trait frequencies — 90
4. Non-metric Post-Cranial trait frequencies — 91
5. Non-metric Dental trait frequencies — 92
6. Non-metric Dental trait frequencies of comparative samples — 96
7. Non-metric Cranial trait frequencies of comparative samples — 98
8. Equations — 99

MAPS
1. Eastern Mediterranean — 101
2. Cyprus — 102
3. Souskiou general area — 103
4. Lemba-Lakkous main area — 104
5. Lemba-Lakkous Area 1 — 105
6. Lemba-Lakkous Area 2 — 106
7. Kissonerga-Mosphilia general area — 107
8. Kissonerga-Mosphilia main area — 108
9. Ayios Iakovos general area — 109
10. Ayios Iakovos drawings of chamber tombs — 110
11. Enkomi general area — 111
12. Enkomi excavated area — 112
13. Asine general area – Barbouna slope and Kastoraki — 113
14. Asine excavated areas — 114
15. Asine Lower Town — 115
16. Lerna general area — 116
17. Lerna excavated area — 117
18. Jerablus-Tahtani excavated area — 118

LIST OF TABLES

Table 2.1:	Sites in study with MNI and time periods	3
Table 2.2:	Radiocarbon dates for Lemba-Lakkous time periods	6
Table 2.3:	Radiocarbon dates for Kissonerga-Mosphilia time periods	7
Table 2.4:	Radiocarbon dates for Ayios Iakovos time periods	8
Table 2.5:	Chronological sequence of cultural phases at Lerna	12
Table 2.6:	Chronological sequence at Jerablus-Tahtani	13
Table 3.1:	Age groups	17
Table 3.2:	Breakdown by sex of all sub-adults and adults from Cyprus	19
Table 4.1:	Combined demography and male-female breakdown of all sites	23
Table 4.2:	Mortality of southwest Cyprus	24
Table 4.3:	Adult Mortality of southwest Cyprus	26
Table 4.4:	Kolmogorov-Smirnov Test for all comparisons	27
Table 4.5:	Mortality of Khirokitia-Vounoi	28
Table 4.6:	Khirokitia-Vounoi Adult Mortality	28
Table 4.7:	Mortality of Jerablus-Tahtani and Karataş-Semayük	30
Table 4.8:	Jerablus-Tahtani and Karataş-Semayük Adult Mortality	32
Table 4.9:	Mortality of Asine, Lerna and Kephala	33
Table 4.10:	Adult Mortality of Asine, Lerna, Kephala and Ayios Kosmas	35
Table 4.11:	Breakdown by sex of adults from Greece	35
Table 4.12:	Mortality of Ayios Iakovos and Enkomi	36
Table 4.13:	Adult Mortality of Ayios Iakovos and Enkomi	37
Table 4.14:	Breakdown by sex of adults from Ayios Iakovos and Enkomi	37
Table 5.1:	Regional stature comparison (cm)	43
Table 5.2:	Cranial non-metric trait frequencies by region	46
Table 5.3:	Post-cranial non-metric trait frequencies by region	47
Table 6.1:	Pair-wise distances (D.θ) between all sites	49
Table 6.2:	Pair-wise distances (D.θ) between all sites	50
Table 6.3:	Pair-wise distances (MMD) between all sites	53
Table 6.4:	Pair-wise distances (MMD)	53
Table 6.5:	Pair-wise distances (D.θ) between regions	57
Table 6.6:	Pair-wise distances (MMD) between regions	59

LIST OF FIGURES

Figure 4.1:	Southwest Cyprus Mortality Profile and E=30	25
Figure 4.2:	Survivorship of southwest Cyprus and E=30	26
Figure 4.3:	Mortality profiles for southwest Cyprus and Khirokitia	29
Figure 4.4:	Survivorship of southwest Cyprus and Khirokitia	29
Figure 4.5:	Mortality of Jerablus-Tahtani, Karataş-Semayük and E=30	31
Figure 4.6:	Survivorship for Jerablus-Tahtani, Karataş-Semayük and E=30	31
Figure 4.7:	Mortality of Asine, Lerna, Kephala and E=30	34
Figure 4.8:	Survivorship for Asine, Lerna, Kephala and E=30	35
Figure 4.9:	Mortality of Enkomi, Ayios Iakovos and E=30	37
Figure 4.10:	Survivorship of northeast Cyprus and E=30	38
Figure 5.1:	Male average stature from combined long bones	41
Figure 5.2:	Female average stature from combined long bones	41
Figure 5.3:	Male and female average stature from all long bones	42
Figure 5.4:	Cranial non-metric trait frequencies by region	45
Figure 6.1:	Tree diagram of the $D.\theta$ means for all sites	51
Figure 6.2:	Multi-dimensional scaling of the $D.\theta$ values from Table 6.1	52
Figure 6.3:	Tree diagram of the MMD means for all sites	54
Figure 6.4:	Multi-dimensional scaling of the MMD values from Table 6.5	55
Figure 6.5:	Dendogram produced by mean linkage hierarchical clustering of the $D.\theta$ values	57
Figure 6.6:	Multi-dimensional scaling of the $D.\theta$ values from Table 6.5	58
Figure 6.7:	Dendogram produced by mean linkage hierarchical clustering of the MMD values	59
Figure 6.8:	Multi-dimensional scaling of the MMD values from Table 6.6	60

ABBREVIATION

Sites

Cyprus
Kissonerga-Mosphilia:	KM
Lemba-Lakkous:	LL
Souskiou:	SOU
Enkomi:	EN
Ayios Iakovos:	AI
Khirokitia:	KHIR

Greece
Asine:	AS
Lerna:	LER
Ayios Kosmas:	AK
Kephala:	KE

Syria
Jerablus-Tahtani:	JT

Turkey
Karataş-Semayük:	KS

Time Periods
Early Bronze Age:	EBA
Middle Bronze Age:	MBA
Late Bronze Age:	LBA
Pre Pottery Neolithic A:	PPNA
Pre Pottery Neolithic B:	PPNB
Early Helladic:	EH
Middle Helladic:	MH
Late Helladic:	LH

Equations and other
Frequency:	p
Mean Measure of Divergence:	MMD
Coefficient of d theta:	$D.\theta$
Average:	Avg
Number:	No.

CHAPTER 1

INTRODUCTION

In the science of archaeology the main focus is usually on the cultural artefacts, which are the predominant remains. It is from this, in which culture, technology, social structure and ideology or religion of a group of people is determined. Even relations and affinities between groups of people are determined using the same evidence. Therefore the spread of human culture has as much to do with the transmission of ideas as is has to do with the transmission of genes. Culture can change regardless of change in biological affinities of a population. In the past, archaeologists have attributed the discovery of a new culture as evidence of a migration of people. However, the spread of ideas need not be related to the movement of genes. Archaeologists examine cultural artefacts, which may have been transmitted by ideas, through communication and trade, rather than an actual arrival of new people (new biological material). The actual individuals (the human remains) of each culture are not considered in this scenario. In the study of physical anthropology, human remains make up an integral part of determining the biological relatedness of people. Traditionally, anthropologists have used cranial metrics, cranial shapes, non-metric traits from the cranial and post-cranial skeleton and dentition in determining the biological affinities of people. More recently, DNA extraction from prehistoric skeletal remains has also been used to identify and relate different groups.

In most cases human remains are found in very poor condition and are often ignored because of the perceived limited information, which can be gained from studying them. The methods used by physical anthropologists all have specific drawbacks when applied to poorly preserved and highly fragmented human remains. While fragmented remains do not affect DNA extraction techniques, they do require strict contamination control protocols to guarantee a successful sample being drawn for analysis. These methods are not possible where these protocols were not observed, nor from older excavations. There is also the added expense of specially trained personnel and expensive equipment needed to carry out the analysis. In comparison, the collection of non-metric traits is an acceptable alternative when the material is very fragmented and in poor condition (Berry & Berry 1967). It can also be used on material from older excavations. This technique can be carried out by personnel with basic anthropological training and does not require special equipment.

1.1 PRINCIPAL AIMS

One of the goals of this study is to identify the biological affinities of various populations from around the eastern Mediterranean, then compare the biological distinctiveness of each group to its neighbours. This will be accomplished primarily by using dental non-metric traits. The skeletal material in this study comes from Greece, Cyprus and Syria, from the Cypriot Chalcolithic to the Late Bronze Age. Non-metric studies have been conducted on other groups but not on the prehistoric people from the countries mentioned above. By combining archaeological and non-metric data, this study will present a holistic approach to studying the people of ancient Cyprus and the eastern Mediterranean.

Another goal of this study is to demonstrate to archaeologists and anthropologists who work in the eastern Mediterranean in which documenting the demographic attributes, health status and biological affinities of all skeletal samples should be included in archaeological reports for all sites. Aegean archaeology in particular has in the past focused primarily on material culture. The physical remains of ancient peoples should be considered as accessible and reliable sources of data to be included in the overall study of ancient civilisations (Alt & Vach 1998; Robb et al. 2001).

The human remains in this study come from eight sites: five in Cyprus, two in Greece and one in Syria. Since 5 out of the 8 sites are from Cyprus, this island will be the main focus of the analysis and discussion with regards to the two different time periods – the Cypriot Chalcolithic and Late Bronze Age. From an archaeological point of view, Cyprus has served as a conduit in the eastern Mediterranean between the civilisations of the east and Europe (Gjerstad et al., 1934). This bridging of ideas and biology makes it an ideal study location to examine the movement of culture and the way the movement of culture and people differ in the spread of human civilisation. This is supported by Dr. Domurad regarding the importance of Cyprus for a regional study of this nature: "Cyprus is particularly well-suited for a population study both because of its location in the eastern Mediterranean, and because it is an island."(Domurad 1986:157). Since the number of sites in this study is limited, the focus on biological relatedness will be between sites rather than changes over time. This study consists of 7 sections:

1. Time Period, Region and Skeletal Samples
2. Anthropological Methods
3. Demography
4. Stature and Non-Metrics
5. Bio-Distance
6. Discussion
7. Conclusion

An important factor to consider regarding this study is not to assume these populations are homogenous. The biological affinities of each site will represent the culmination of cultural, geographical and genetic effects over a large period of time. The data collected will only represent a cross section of each site at the time of the deposition of the human remains.

One of the arguments presented in this study is movement of culture does not always indicate the movement of people. It is assumed in distance studies people closer in geographical distance will be close in biological affinities (Buikstra et al 1990). This is also the case for people with similar or overlapping cultures. This thesis will argue this cannot be assumed until the human remains are actually studied in order to demonstrate the relationship. Time is also a factor in interpreting the relationship between different groups. Trade, technology (sea-faring or other transportation technology) or social and religious factors, which are very difficult to determine, can also affect the transmission of ideas and biology.

1.2 ARCHAEOLOGICAL QUESTIONS

The limited samples in this study somewhat restrict which questions can be addressed. Therefore specific questions will be addressed to the different regions the samples are from. The main focus of the archaeological questions will revolve around Cyprus, specifically the southwest Chalcolithic part of the island since most of the samples are from there. The lack of any previous dental non-metric analysis from these sites permits me to address the following questions on the biological make-up of these sites:

1. Does Chalcolithic Cyprus represent a homogeneous biological as well as cultural group (all three sites belong to the Erimi culture)?
2. Is the there a difference between the biological affinities of village versus cemetery sites in Chalcolithic Cyprus? Since Souskiou-Vathyrkakas represents the only cemetery from Cyprus is there a biological distribution difference between the settlements of Lemba-Lakkous and Kissonerga-Mosphilia with the cemetery, which have some different burial practices?
3. What social implications do these similarities or differences have to understanding Chalcolithic Cyprus?
4. Do the sites in northeast Late Bronze Age Cyprus represent a homogeneous biological as well as cultural group?
5. Do the sites in Late Bronze Age Cyprus share any biological continuity with Chalcolithic Cyprus?
6. Do the sites in Middle Bronze Age Greece represent a homogeneous biological as well as cultural group?

These questions will be addressed mainly within the context of the dental non-metric traits, but also in conjunction with the demographic evidence. The archaeological data will also be taken into account when discussing these questions.

1.3 METHOD

Standard anthropological data will be collected and analysed in this study along with the non-metric traits. The data will be used in a demographic analysis between the sites and will also be compared to other samples. The non-metric data from each site will be analysed with the use of two distance equations, the Mean Measure of Divergence (MMD) and the Coefficient of θ ($D.\theta$). As there is no comparable non-metric data from the eastern Mediterranean from the time periods in this study, data from geographically close samples will have to be included as a comparison to my samples. This data will also be compared to other non-metric samples from various time periods from the Epipalaeolithic to the Bronze Age and from the Levant to northern Europe.

This study will also take into account how the biological affinities relate to the archaeological data from each site. The data will be used not only to address the specific questions above but will also be presented to assist the understanding of the cultural context between the samples.

CHAPTER 2

TIME PERIOD, REGION AND SKELETAL SAMPLES

2.1 INTRODUCTION

This study examined the skeletal remains of 786 individuals from eight prehistoric sites around the eastern Mediterranean (Table 2.1). The samples are from three geographical areas: Greece, Syria and Cyprus (Map 1). Table 2.1 lists each site and its time period. Appendix 1 places all sites into a regional chronology.

The selection of sites in this study was mainly based on the availability of sufficiently large skeletal assemblages. Many smaller assemblages in Greece and in Cyprus were available but a minimum of 40 individuals was necessary for the dental non-metric and for the demographic analyses. Great effort was made to include skeletal assemblages from Turkey, in order to have an adequate regional comparison, but no one responded to my correspondence. The skeletal collection from Turkey, which would have been ideal for this study, is the large assemblage from the Early Bronze cemetery of Karataş-Semayük (Angel 1968; 1970). It was not possible to study this assemblage personally. There were other smaller samples from the sites of İkiztepe (Becker 1988), Kurban Höyük (Alpagut 1986) and Şeyh Höyük (Şenyürek and Tunakan 1951; Şenyürek 1955) which I was not able to gain access to. These samples are too small to be adequate for dental non-metric analysis. There were also no comparative data on dental non-metrics available from Turkey which could be included.

Archaeological data from the sites have already been published, with the exception of Jerablus-Tahtani and Souskiou-Vathyrkakas for which only preliminary reports have been published. The following section presents a brief summary of the sites, including specific aspects of cultural and archaeological data. More detailed information on the sites presented is available in the published reports.

The following list of selected archaeological data will be followed by a brief summary for each country. Cyprus has been divided into Chalcolithic southwest Cyprus and Late Bronze Age northeast Cyprus since the cultures are different.

Country	Site	MNI	Time Period
Cyprus	Souskiou (SOU)	38	Chalcolithic
	Lemba-Lakkous (LL)	52	Chalcolithic/Early Bronze
	Kissonerga-Mosphilia (KM)	78	Chalcolithic/Early Bronze
	Ayios Iakovos (AI)	45	Late Bronze
	Enkomi (EN)	76	Late Bronze
Greece	Asine (AS)	145	Middle Bronze
	Lerna (LER)	229	Middle Bronze
Syria	Jerablus-Tahtani (JT)	123	Early Bronze
Total		786	

Table 2.1 – Sites in study with MNI and time periods

2.2 CYPRUS:
INTRODUCTION

The island of Cyprus yielded an interesting collection of sites for this study. The five Cypriot sites encompass the greatest time span. The occupation of these sites begins in the Cypriot Chalcolithic and spans the whole duration of the Bronze Age. From an archaeological point of view, Cyprus has served as a connecting point between the cultures and perhaps genes of east and west (Gjerstad et al., 1934). This bridging of ideas and biology makes it an ideal study location to examine the movement of culture and to understand the way the movement of culture and people differ in the spread of human civilisation.

2.2.1 SOUSKIOU
2.2.1.1 LOCATION

The site of Souskiou is located in the southwest of Cyprus in the Paphos District (Map 2). Souskiou is a series of three cemeteries all in the same area, called Laona, Vathyrkakas 1 and 2. The three cemeteries are located between the abandoned village of Souskiou and the modern village of Kouklia (Maier & Karageorghis 1984; Niklasson 1991; Maier & Wartburg 1994). The skeletal remains studied were only from Vathyrkakas 1 and 2. These skeletal remains are stored at the Lemba Archaeological centre, the University of Edinburgh and the University of Glasgow.

2.2.1.2 SETTING

Souskiou-Vathyrkakas (hereafter Souskiou) is situated on the edge of a plateau, approximately 100m in elevation, bordering the deep ravine, which leads off from the river Diarrhizos which runs to the north (Map 3) (Maier 1973; Stanley Price 1980). The cemetery is a roughly rectangular shaped area, measuring approximately 50m by 15m (Niklasson 1991). The supposed settlement site near the cemetery is called Laona (Hadjisavvas 1977). This small area has been inhabited from Neolithic up to medieval times. A possible reason for such a long occupation was the abundance of water in the area (Hadjisavvas 1977). The cemeteries were found at a height ranging from 150 to 180 metres above sea level (Hadjisavvas 1977).

2.2.1.3 HISTORY

Souskiou is a unique site with a long and somewhat complicated excavation history. The site has been known since the 1950's and has yielded much information about Cypriot Chalcolithic burial customs (Niklasson 1991). In 1950 the British Kouklia expedition led by T. B. Mitford and J. H. Iliffe made a four-week long investigation in the area of Palaeopaphos (Mitford & Iliffe 1951; Christou 1989; Niklasson 1991). They discovered the Vathyrkakas cemetery 1, with "…a multitude of tombs, for the most part long since looted" (Mitford & Iliffe 1951). The following year, three undisturbed graves were excavated which uncovered Red-on-White (RW) pottery and dentalium necklaces with cruciform picrolite pendants (Niklasson 1991). In 1972, 17 rock cut tombs were looted in cemetery 1 and a Swiss-German excavation directed by F.-G. Maier worked on the looted graves to save as much evidence as possible (Maier 1973; Niklasson 1991; Maier & Wartburg 1994). The Swiss-German excavation also located Vathyrkakas 2, situated approximately 400 m west of cemetery 1, and found at least 14 looted and emptied graves (Niklasson 1991; Maier & Wartburg 1994).

The excavations of the Cyprus Department of Antiquities on Cemetery 1, led by D. Christou from December 4 to 10, 1972, located another 5 graves (Christou 1989; Niklasson 1991). A settlement site of the same date, Laona, situated on an isolated spur of land opposite the cemeteries, was at the same time identified by Maier's team. Here, a fair amount of RW sherds were seen on the surface, but no buildings were located (Maier 1973; Niklasson 1991).

Conducting a large scale survey in the Paphos District in 1975, S. Hadjisavvas discovered a third cemetery, called Laona, situated approximately 250 m NE of the Laona settlement site (Hadjisavvas 1977). Together with a few RW sherds, an undetermined number of looted graves were also identified (Hadjisavvas 1977; Niklasson 1991).

Between 1991 and 1997 a rescue excavation was conducted on Souskiou-Vathyrkakas 1 and 2 by the Department of Antiquities, which exposed 50-70 extra tombs, some of which were included in this study.

2.2.1.4 TIME PERIOD

The cemeteries are dated to the Cypriot Middle Chalcolithic (Chalcolithic II) (c. 4000-3500 BC) (Christou 1989). The predominance of RW ware and an absence of Combed and Red Polished ware point to a Chalcolithic I date (Maier 1973). The three cemeteries, Souskiou-Vathyrkakas 1 and 2 and Laona, are probably contemporary with Erimi levels (Niklasson 1991). The cruciform figurines and pendants from the sites also suggest similarities to examples from Erimi and Kythrea, which fall into the second phase of the Erimi culture (approximately 3600 BC) (Christou 1989).

2.2.1.5 TYPE OF SITE

Souskiou is the earliest recorded cemetery in western Cyprus (Peltenburg 1985a). This site is unique for the Chalcolithic time period on Cyprus because all known Neolithic and Chalcolithic burials have always been found beneath or very near the people's houses. The settlement at Souskiou in comparison is quite a distance away (Maier 1973). According to Maier, there is enough evidence to support the theory these three cemeteries are related to the nearby settlement (Maier 1973).

2.2.1.6 LOCATION, TYPE AND NUMBER OF TOMBS

As the cemetery is some distance from the settlement, which has been identified, these tombs are to be considered extramural (Niklasson 1991). The tombs in all three cemeteries are bottle-shaped (or bell-shaped) pits or shafts (Type I) entirely cut into the hard limestone rock (Peltenburg 1979; Niklasson 1991). Type II graves are simple upper rock cut pits (Niklasson 1991). This type of tomb is unique in Cyprus and it differs considerably from the contemporary tombs at Erimi in the Limassol district, which are much larger than the pit-shaped tombs of Lemba-Lakkous (Maier & Karageorghis 1984). Dimensions of most tombs (rock cut pits) are Length 1.00-1.60 m, Width 0.50-0.90 and Depth 1.45-2.20 m (L and W concern the mouths of the pits) (Niklasson 1991). The tombs were filled with soil and covered with capstones, many of which were found during excavation (Peltenburg 1979; Maier & Karageorghis 1984; Christou 1989).

Twenty-five tombs are known from Vathyrkakas Cemetery 1, 14 from Vathyrkakas Cemetery 2, and an unknown number from Laona. According to Niklasson, the total number of graves should exceed at least 50 (Niklasson 1991). A total of 38 individuals from only 15 tombs were studied during the course of this research, which is majority of human remains reported by Niklasson (1991).

The tombs are primary burials with no evidence of secondary burial activity. All of the tombs held more than one individual. The deceased were buried at the bottom in a contracted position, as in the Neolithic period, accompanied by rich grave goods (Peltenburg 1979; Maier & Karageorghis 1984; Christou 1989). According to Christou (1989) the orientation of the graves at Vathyrkakas is east west with a tendency towards northwest southeast.

Peltenburg notes the uniqueness of Souskiou for the Chalcolithic in which three rich cemeteries, all located in a very small area, for one small settlement seems excessive (Peltenburg 1979; 1982b). Peltenburg speculates the cemeteries could be part of a boundary site, on the frontier between districts and they may be special burial grounds for a regional population rather than simply for the adjacent village (pers. comm. E. Peltenburg).

2.2.1.7 GRAVE GOODS

As there has been extensive looting at the site, some of the grave goods have been purchased from dealers. Therefore, the provenience of some artefacts is in dispute. A number of artefacts, however, have been recovered from the excavation. Many picrolite cruciform figurines and pendants have been recovered from the tombs, as well as Red-on-White pottery (Christou 1989). These cruciform figurines are unique to western Cyprus during the Chalcolithic (Peltenburg 1979). A copper ornament with a spiral design has also been recovered, which represents only the second copper object found in the Cypriot Chalcolithic (Christou 1989). Necklaces and picrolite cruciform figurines appear to have been the most common artefact found in the tombs at Souskiou-Vathyrkakas (Vagnetti 1980; Peltenburg 1985a).

The main pottery type found in the tombs and at the settlement is Red-on-White (RW) ceramic ware (Maier 1973; Maier & Karageorghis 1984; Christou 1989). The RW style is also known from other Chalcolithic sites such as Erimi (Maier & Karageorghis 1984). Mostly bowls and some bottle shapes have been found (Maier & Karageorghis 1984), and terracotta zoomorphic figurines (Peltenburg 1990; Niklasson 1991).

2.2.2 LEMBA-LAKKOUS
2.2.2.1 LOCATION

Lemba-Lakkous (hereafter Lemba) is located in the northern part of the Ktima Lowlands about 4 km north of Paphos in southwestern Cyprus (Map 4). The settlement sits between an unnamed stream and the Agriokalami River (Peltenburg 1985a). The site is roughly 1000m from the coast with an elevation of approximately 60m (Stanley Price 1980). The skeletal remains are stored at the Museum of Paphos.

2.2.2.2 SETTING

The Ktima Lowlands consist of a coastal strip some 25 km long and a maximum of 11 km wide, from Kissonerga to Kouklia with Paphos near its mid-point. The terrain is characterised by a series of sea terraces, which are crossed by small streams (Peltenburg 1985a).

Presently, fishing and the rearing of livestock play a small role in the subsistence of the local inhabitants. Most of the current settlements are not situated along the coast (Kato-Paphos is the exception). The local water supply is based on perennial spring flow, which is affected by climate change (Peltenburg 1985a). Studies on the palaeo-climate and palaeobotanical assemblages show little evidence that present day Cyprus is much different from ancient Cyprus (Peltenburg 1985a).

2.2.2.3 HISTORY

The site of Lemba was first surveyed by Sophocles Hadjisavvas (1977), who conducted a detailed survey and test excavation between 1975 and 1976. Under the direction of E. Peltenburg of the University of Edinburgh, excavations began in 1976 until 1983, with a total of 7 seasons of excavations. According to Peltenburg (Peltenburg 1985a), one of the goals of the Lemba Archaeological Project was to understand the nature of change in society, in this case, the fundamental differences between the Sotira and Erimi groups and between the Erimi and Early Cypriot Period.

> "Cyprus, being an island, is ideally placed for the study of such an issue. Its history might well be described as one of punctuated equilibrium, that is long periods of homeostasis interrupted by relatively short spells in which change occurs." (Peltenburg 1985a:1)

To address the problem of studying many short-lived sites, the Lemba Archaeological Project had to be a regional survey combined with localised multi-site excavations. There is a Cypriot phenomenon, during this time period, of short-lived villages where there is abandonment and then resettlement, most likely to nearby locations (Peltenburg 1985a).

2.2.2.4 TIME PERIOD OF SITE

The occupation of the settlement mostly takes place during the Chalcolithic and ends during the Early Bronze Age and is part of the Erimi culture as is Souskiou. The following radiocarbon dates are all from charcoal (Table 2.2) (Peltenburg 1985a). Period 3 is the most securely dated period of the three. According to Peltenburg the charcoal radiocarbon dates support rather than contradict the proposed ceramic dating of the site (Peltenburg 1985a). The human remains come from tombs throughout all three of the time periods, although most are from the last 2 periods.

Period	Radiocarbon dates	Calibrated BC dates	Period
1	5000±260	3500-3000	Middle Chalcolithic
2	3930±100	3400-2800	Middle Chalcolithic
3	4050±50	2700-2400	Late Chalcolithic

Table 2.2 – Radiocarbon dates of Lemba-Lakkous time periods (Radiocarbon dates from Peltenburg 1985a:16)

2.2.2.5 TYPE OF SITE

Lemba-Lakkous is a small village approximately 3 ha in size. Prehistoric Cyprus is usually characterised by single-period sites, while the evidence of two ceramic groups from Lemba suggests it is a multi-period site (Peltenburg 1985a). Two major areas of occupation were excavated, Areas I and II, which are approximately 100 m apart (Niklasson 1991). With the aid of ceramics as well as radio-carbon dating and what little stratigraphic information was available, three periods of occupation have been determined (Niklasson 1991).

The majority of evidence comes from Period 1, Area 1 (Map 5) (Peltenburg 1985a). Period 3 seems to be represented in Area II and seems to be the period of the most building activity (Map 6). The problem of stratigraphy suggests an interrupted occupation with a break between Periods 1 and 2 and possibly between Periods 2 and 3 (Niklasson 1991). The houses are sub-circular, approximately 3 m in diameter, built with stone and pisé (rammed earth floors), covered walls, and most have multiple occupation phases (Peltenburg 1985a; Peltenburg 1990).

2.2.2.6 LOCATION, TYPE AND NUMBER OF TOMBS

Fifty-six graves containing sixty individuals have been excavated, which at the time was the largest number of burials from a Chalcolithic site in Cyprus. Of these, twenty-two graves were found in Area I and thirty-four in Area II (Peltenburg 1985a). A possible further fourteen graves were discovered and excavated without any skeletal remains found (Niklasson 1991).

The graves are mainly intramural (under and around the houses and within the village boundary) but other cemeteries from this time period, such as Souskiou and Kouklia, are extramural (graves from Erimi and Karavas are intramural like at Lemba) (Peltenburg 1985a). Primary burials predominate, but there is evidence approximately fifteen individuals received secondary burials. Predominately these 15 are children and infants (Niklasson 1991).

There are two types of graves. Type I is a simple pit grave and type II are burial pits situated below a shallow, roughly circular upper pit (whereby a capstone could be put in place)(Peltenburg 1985a). The grave types here have structural elements from Erimi and Souskiou as well as new ones (Peltenburg et al. 1979). The graves are predominately single interments with only four graves having two or even up to four infants (Peltenburg 1985a). Evidence from the undisturbed burials suggests the deceased were mainly placed in a contracted position (Niklasson 1991). Most of the graves were orientated north south with some variations such as three graves with an east-west orientation (Niklasson 1991). Individuals were usually placed on their right side in a crouched position with their hands to the northeast facing their heads (Peltenburg et al. 1979).

It is not known whether the extra human remains in some tombs represent reused tombs (Peltenburg 1985a). The reuse of existing graves has also occurred at the Neolithic sites of Khirokitia and Cap Andreas Kastros (Dikaios 1953), with a true double burial recently discovered at Kissonerga-Mosphilia (Peltenburg 1985a). It is not known whether the people of Lemba-Lakkous buried their dead in family graves or familial areas, but three infants buried just southeast of Building 12 could be related (Peltenburg 1985a).

2.2.2.7 GRAVE GOODS

Very few grave goods were found in Area I or II (other than picrolite pendants and necklaces) and most were found with children and young people (Niklasson 1985). One of the pendants appears to have been worn during the lifetime of the child and there is evidence it had been repaired in antiquity. This could suggest these objects were made not only for funerary purposes, but were pendants people wore during life (Peltenburg 1985a).

2.2.3 KISSONERGA-MOSPHILIA
2.2.3.1 LOCATION

Kissonerga-Mosphilia (hereafter Mosphilia) is located in southwestern Cyprus, situated 6 km north of Paphos in the Ktima lowlands on the coastal plain below the village of Kissonerga-Mosphilia. The site is approximately 500 m from the present shoreline on the N side of the Skotinis River and 1.5 km north of Lemba-Lakkous (Map 7) (Peltenburg et al. 1998). The skeletal remains are stored at the Museum of Paphos.

2.2.3.2 SETTING

The site is 1.5 km north of Lemba-Lakkous and so is in a similar setting to the previous site. Just as with Lemba-Lakkous, there are no obvious outstanding natural features to account for the location or longevity of the site (Peltenburg et al. 1998). The Skotinis stream forms the southern edge of the site.

The site has an irregular oval shape 300 x 500 m and an elevation of approximately 40m above sea level (Stanley Price 1980). The area of the site is approximately 12 ha, and it is the largest Chalcolithic site in the Ktima lowlands. This site follows the pattern for prehistoric Cyprus, where settlements are abandoned for some time and then reoccupied (Peltenburg et al. 1998).

2.2.3.3 HISTORY

The first person to report on the existence of the prehistoric site at Mosphilia was A.H.S. Megaw (Megaw 1952; Peltenburg et al. 1998). In 1971 E. Peltenburg and N. Stanley Price visited the site and in 1975 S. Hadjisavvas (1977) made a detailed survey of the area. Some exceptional pieces found at the site include a picrolite cruciform figurine, a stone bowl fragment and Middle Bronze Age pottery. The excavation of the site which is part of the Lemba Archaeological Project under the direction of E. Peltenburg of the University of Edinburgh began in 1979 and lasted until 1992, with a total of six seasons of excavations plus survey work (Peltenburg et al. 1998).

2.2.3.4 TIME PERIOD

The time period of the site is from the Cypriot Neolithic until slightly past the end of the Chalcolithic. The site is also part of the Erimi cultural group. The following dates are all from charcoal radiocarbon dates (Table 2.3 Modified from fig 2.3) (Peltenburg et al. 1998).

Period	Radiocarbon dates	Calibrated BC dates	Period
1A	7,255±60 BP	6000	Neolithic
2	5,320±90 – 4,860±80 BP	4000-3800	Early Chalcolithic
3A	5,540±110 – 4,285±60 BP	3500-3100	Middle Chalcolithic
3A/4	4,020±110 BP	3200	Middle Chalcolithic
3B	4,690±70 – 3,880±100 BP	3000-2900	Middle Chalcolithic
3 / 4	4,170±80 BP	3000-2700	Middle Chalcolithic
4	5,620±3,900±50 BP	2400-2700	Late Chalcolithic
5	3,900±50 BP	2500	Philia culture

Table 2.3 – Radiocarbon dates from the time periods from Mosphilia

2.2.3.5 TYPE OF SITE

Mosphilia is a small village, with some purpose-built storage facilities and some mortuary structures. Most houses are circular and some rectangular (Map 8) (Peltenburg et al. 1998). Mosphilia was a wealthy and long-lived village. Building 3 was filled with a vast array of stacked pithoi, indicating collection, storage and perhaps redistribution at the end of the period (Bolger 1989). The large size of the site could also suggest it was an important ceremonial site (Niklasson 1991).

2.2.3.6 LOCATION, TYPE AND NUMBER OF TOMBS

The burials are located within the settlement and are mostly found under or beside the houses (Peltenburg et al. 1998). There are 5 grave types from the period 3A to 5, in which human remains have been located:

1. Pit Graves
2. Pit Graves with caps
3. Chamber tombs
4. Pot burials
5. Scoop grave

Grave types 1 and 2 are mainly used in period 3A and 3B, while period 4 shows some use of grave types 1 and 2, as well as a greater use of grave types 3 and 5. Period 5, which has the least number of burials, only has type 4 graves

(Peltenburg et al. 1998). Also in period 4, there is a feature, which is referred to as Mortuary Enclosure B357. It is a circular wall of posts of unknown dimensions. The mortuary structure held 9 individuals and since it does not share any of the features of the houses, it is thought to be a special burial area (Peltenburg et al. 1998).

2.2.3.7 GRAVE GOODS

The artefacts found in the tombs are relatively few compared to later Early Bronze Age burials (Peltenburg et al. 1998). The types of artefacts range from various types of pottery, picrolite pendants and figurines, and faience beads to stone and bone objects (Peltenburg et al. 1998). The specific types of artefacts are not as important for this study as are the changes in type and distribution of artefacts, which occur at the site.

The difference occurs between Period 3B and 4, first with regards to the great number of picrolite pendants found with children in period 3B. In Period 4 there is a shift in child burials from multiple interments with grave goods to single burials with few grave goods (Peltenburg et al. 1998). Special production of ceramic funerary goods is introduced in Period 4. Peltenburg also mentions in Period 4 Anatolian-influenced pouring vessels are found only with adult burials and within the Mortuary Enclosure suggesting a possible elite group in the society (Peltenburg et al. 1998). Another change in Period 4 is the appearance of Red-and-Black Stroke-Burnished ware (RB/B), which dominates the assemblage.

2.2.4 AYIOS IAKOVOS
2.2.4.1 LOCATION

The site is located in the northeastern part of Cyprus. The village of Ayios Iakovos is located approximately 22.5 km north of Famagusta (Gjerstad et al. 1934; Åström 1966). The tombs are situated 1.5 km east of the village of Ayios Iakovos, in the locality of Melia (Map 9). To the west there is a small region of pine trees and the village of Mandre is located 1.8 km north at the foot of the Kerynia Mountains (Gjerstad et al. 1934). The skeletal remains are stored at the University of Göteborg, Sweden and the Museum of Near East Studies in Stockholm, Sweden.

2.2.4.2 SETTING

The area with the tombs is a relatively flat, poorly cultivated plain of limestone rock and sand. According to Gjerstad et al. (1934), the homogeneous nature of the rock created an ideal condition for the tomb builders to cut the tomb chambers without interference.

2.2.4.3 HISTORY

This site was excavated as part of the Swedish Expedition to Cyprus for 3½ years from September 1927 to March 1931 (Gjerstad et al. 1934). Fourteen tombs were excavated in the seven weeks of the Swedish expedition uncovering a total of approximately 40 individuals (Fischer 1986). Some of these tombs had suffered from illegal excavations in the past. Another excavation was carried out for 2 days in 1959 by Paul Åström, uncovered another chamber tomb (No. 15). The remains from this tomb have not been included in this study (Åström 1966).

2.2.4.4 TIME PERIOD

From the 14 tombs excavated, only tombs 8 and 14 have been studied. These tombs date from Middle Cycladic IIIC to Late Cycladic IIA (Gjerstad et al. 1934) (Table 2.4). The date of Tomb 8 is the later half of the Middle Cycladic III period but most of the contents and the burials are from the Late Cycladic period (Gjerstad et al. 1934).

Time Period	Tombs	Dates
MC III C	8	1725-1600 BC
LC I A	8	1600-1450 BC
LC II A	8, 14	1450-1200 BC

Table 2.4 – Radiocarbon dates for the time periods from Ayios Iakovos (From Åström 1966)

2.2.4.5 TYPE OF SITE

No settlement was located therefore the site is an extramural cemetery (Gjerstad et al. 1934; Åström 1966).

2.4.4.6 LOCATION, TYPE AND NUMBER OF TOMBS

When I traveled to the University of Göteborg to study the remains, I was only able to locate remains from tombs 8 and 14 totaling approximately 30 individuals. Peter Fischer (1986), who studied all the remains from the Swedish excavation, refers to other individuals, which could not be located at the University of Göteborg. Therefore I have included the remaining data, which Fischer studied, in my demographic analysis (but not any dental non-metric data).

These tombs are Late Bronze Age rock cut and stone-built, large chamber tombs, very well made and held many people. The tombs also had a dromos that led down to the chamber (Map 10) (Gjerstad et al. 1934). Tombs 8 and 13 seem to show evidence of multiple period burials with as many as 60 people buried in the tombs at different times. All of the tombs were sealed with capstones. No coffins were used; the bodies were extended in a dorsal position (Gjerstad et al. 1934).

2.2.4.7 GRAVE GOODS

Most of the goods found in the tombs were ceramics: black slip I-II ware, white painted and Red-on-Black wares (Gjerstad et al. 1934). Some plain hand-made ware, mixed with red polished IV, while red slip and black on red wares were also found in the tombs (Gjerstad et al., 1934).

2.2.5 ENKOMI
2.2.5.1 LOCATION

Enkomi is located in the northeastern Cyprus approximately 18 km east of the cemetery of Ayios Iakovos (Map 11) (Gjerstad et al. 1934). The skeletal remains are stored at the University of Göteborg, Sweden and the Museum of Near East Studies in Stockholm, Sweden.

2.2.5.2 SETTING

The cemetery is close to the present village of Enkomi, approximately 10 km from Famagusta. The site is also known for being an important city for trade during the Late Bronze Age (Åström 1969). The area was reported poorly cultivated scrubland and used mainly as pasture (Gjerstad et al. 1934). The landscape at the necropolis is a white limestone rock, which extends around the area. This area slopes down to a small riverbed (Gjerstad et al. 1934).

2.2.5.3 HISTORY

The site was first found and investigated in 1896 by Murry, Smith and Christian for the Cyprus Exploration Fund (Gjerstad et al. 1934). Since its discovery, the site has been subject to illegal excavation with hundreds of tombs looted. Two separate excavations by the Cyprus Museum in 1913 and by Mr. R. Gunnis in 1927 proved unable to locate any more tombs. The site was part of the Swedish Expedition to Cyprus for 3½ years from September 1927 to March 1931. The tombs discovered were excavated in June and July 1930 (Gjerstad et al. 1934).

2.2.5.4 TIME PERIOD

The tombs are almost all from the Late Cypriot (LC) period, ranging from the LC II-III, with only Tomb 12 (skull FCE 36) being older from Middle Cypriot III (Fischer 1986).

2.2.5.5 TYPE OF SITE

Unlike Ayios Iakovos, the settlement for Enkomi has been located (Åström 1969). Therefore it is a cemetery connected with a large city. A wall once surrounded the necropolis, which is still visible in some places (Map 12) (Gjerstad et al. 1934).

2.2.5.6 LOCATION, TYPE AND NUMBER OF TOMBS

While visiting the University of Göteborg to study the remains I was not able to locate material from all of the tombs, which were excavated. From the approximately 75 individuals mentioned by Fischer (1986), I was only able to study skeletal remains from 65 individuals.

As with Ayios Iakovos, the tombs are large rock cut chambers, but these were dug deeper into the earth than those at Ayios Iakovos (approximately 2 m deep). The nature of the area and the limestone probably made this type of tomb the easiest and most efficient (Gjerstad et al., 1934). All of the tombs were sealed with capstones (Åström 1969). Most of the bodies in these tombs were either lying on their backs extended or sitting up. Exceptions to this are from Tombs 17 where 4 out of the 5 bodies were all found in the traditional Cypriot custom in seated positions (Gjerstad et al. 1934). Multiple burial levels have been recorded for these tombs.

2.2.5.7 GRAVE GOODS

Most of the goods found in the tombs were ceramics, with the exceptions of Tombs 17 and 18 in which some ivory, other metal objects and jewelry were also found. Tomb 18 was the wealthiest tomb excavated with a large amount of imported Levanto-Helladic ware (Gjerstad et al. 1934).

2.2.6 SUMMARY
2.2.6.1 CHALCOLITHIC CYPRUS

Although there are some similarities between the three sites there are some differences. For example, the characteristic picrolite cruciform figurines and burials and the Red-on-While (RW) pottery have been found associated with burials. These two features help to relate these sites to other Erimi sites. The differences between the sites should be noted: Lemba and Mosphilia are villages albeit of different sizes (Mosphilia is much larger), while Souskiou is a cemetery with a small, unexcavated settlement associated with it. The locations of the sites are also different. Lemba and Mosphilia are located on open plains near the coast while Souskiou is located on a high rock outcrop. An obvious difference between the three sites is that Souskiou is a cemetery while Lemba and Mosphilia are villages with burials under the houses. There are some similarities regarding burial practices. The pit and bell/bottle shaped tombs covered with a capstone are found at Souskiou and Lemba while Mosphilia has a range of tomb types from simple pits to more elaborate chamber tombs. Souskiou and Mosphilia also have many more multiple burials while Lemba has mostly single interments.

2.2.6.2 LATE BRONZE AGE

The two Late Bronze sites are very similar overall with both having large multi-period rock cut chamber tombs holding many individuals. While Ayios Iakovos does not have a settlement associated with the necropolis, Enkomi does. They even share similar type of grave goods with black slip I-II ware, white painted, Red-on-Black wares and some plain hand-made ware. Enkomi had some more exotic grave goods along with a large amount of imported Levanto-Helladic ware.

2.3 GREECE:

The two sites from Greece in this study are both from the Middle Bronze Age in the Argolid, in the Peloponnese in southern mainland Greece. Temporally these sites fall between the earliest sites on Cyprus and the latest. They will be used as a comparison for Cyprus from a western perspective.

2.3.1 ASINE
2.3.1.1 LOCATION

The site of Asine is located on the north shore of the Gulf of Argos, approximately 1 km from the modern seaside town of Tolon and approximately 8 km from Nauplion (Map 13) (Nordquist 1987). The human skeletal remains are stored at the University of Uppsala, Sweden.

2.3.1.2 SETTING

The main part of the Middle Helladic (MH) settlement was found on the northwest slope of the rocky outcrop (promontory) known as Kastraki, on the north beach of the Argos Gulf. On Kastraki itself, many ancient remains have been lost due to erosion and human activity (Nordquist 1987). The Lower Town (LT) is on the lower slope of the Barbouna hill and possibly extends out to the plain (Nordquist 1987). On the Barbouna slope, two late MH houses were found and a late MH/early LH extramural cemetery. At least one MH cist-grave and some walls were reported from further to the east, close to the beach (Nordquist 1987). The climate of the LBA Aegean was not greatly different from that of today, other than being a little more arid with higher surface temperatures (Nordquist 1987).

2.3.1.3 HISTORY

The Swedish Expedition to Greece excavated the site between 1922 and 1930 by Otto Frödin and Axel W. Persson (Frödin & Persson 1938; Nordquist & Hägg 1996). The Swedish team excavated for five seasons between 1922 and 1930. The excavation in 1922 began with the acropolis (Kastraki) (Map 14). This campaign uncovered EBA remains in four principal locations: Pre-Mycenaean Terrace, Polygonal Wall, Lower Town and Terrace III (Frödin and Persson 1938). Another excavation in the 1970's by Inga Hägg and Robin Hägg excavated the Middle Helladic settlement and graves on the Barbouna slope (Nordquist & Hägg 1996).

2.3.1.4 TIME PERIOD

The site had been settled as early as the EH and continued to be inhabited through the Bronze Age. By the MH (Middle Bronze Age) it had become the dominant site in the Area (Nordquist 1987). The tombs found mainly date to Early Helladic and Hellenistic periods but also Late Helladic and Geometric artefacts have been discovered (Nordquist 1987).

2.3.1.5 TYPE OF SITE

The site can possibly be considered a small town, playing an important role in the region. The main part of the site was the Lower Terrace (LT) (Map 15). The location of the site on the northwest slope with the hill behind and the Kastraki in front offered some protection against the sun and the winds (Nordquist 1987). The Kastraki probably acted as an acropolis, offering refuge during times of unrest as well as a lookout point for fishing and shipping (Map 14). From my own observations from the top of the Kastraki, there is a view of 360° all around, with the plain to the southeast, the sea to the southwest and the Barbouna slope to the northwest.

There is no evidence of MH fortifications on the Kastraki, possibly because the sea may have isolated it. The connection with the mainland would have been over a bridge or by boat. The acropolis showed little sign of habitation in the MH but more in the EH, used mainly as a lookout and place of refuge with temporary houses built (Nordquist 1987). The burials on the acropolis are considered intramural (Nordquist 1987).

The size of the site (excluding the extramural cemeteries) during the MH period can be roughly estimated to be 1½-2 ha. A similar population density, as with Lerna, has been assumed for Asine, this would suggest a population of 285-399 persons on 1½ ha or 380-532 persons on 2 ha (about 50-93 households) (Nordquist 1987). According to Nordquist:

"It was this combination of access to different resources, agricultural and coastal, in combination with its strategic placing, that gave the site its status and enabled it to survive periods of crisis. Unlike Lerna, it continued to be used all through the LH period, perhaps because it lay some distance from the other centres, but did not develop into a major palace site." (Nordquist 1987:26)

The natural features of the land determined the site planning. With no dedicated planning of the site, it developed 'organically' free standing houses being added when needed and demolished when no longer in use (Nordquist 1987).

2.3.1.6 LOCATION, TYPE AND NUMBER OF TOMBS

East of the acropolis and on the Barbouna slope, an extramural cemetery was found (Nordquist 1987). Asine is a multi-period site with tombs from various times, with cist, pithoi, shaft and simple earth-cut graves (Frödin & Persson 1938). MH graves have been found in all three areas of Asine (Lower Town, Barbouna slope and eastern side of the Kastraki). From the excavations, at least 147 MH graves with approximately 158 individuals have been found (Nordquist 1987).

The absence of walls makes it difficult to distinguish the extramural and intramural cemeteries (Nordquist 1987). The graves in the LT will be considered as an intramural cemetery while the other two will be treated as extramural (Nordquist 1987). The graves of the E cemetery are considered extramural because they are clearly outside the settlement. On the Barbouna slope the houses were destroyed in MH IIIA, and the nearby cemetery spread into the area where the houses had been (Nordquist 1987).

The most common type of tomb throughout the MH was the earth-cut pit grave. They were used for children as well as adults and for both sexes (Nordquist 1987). The MH graves from Asine were orientated NE-SW with the heads usually lying in a northwest or northeast direction, with the skeleton usually laid contracted on the right side (Frödin & Persson 1938).

The tomb designs were three types of stone-built cist-graves: Cist I was the orthostat cist, Cist II had walls constructed of courses of horizontally placed slabs, and Cist III was a mixture of both the other types. Each type was used for both sexes and all ages.

2.3.1.7 GRAVE GOODS

Most of the MH tombs did not have any grave goods (Frödin & Persson 1938; Nordquist 1987). The grave goods which have been found are very basic but with much variety: some matt-painted pottery, shell, obsidian flakes, arrow heads, fish vertebrae and bones of small animals, bronze tweezers and a Yellow Minyan vase (Frödin & Persson 1938; Nordquist 1987).

2.3.2 LERNA
2.3.2.1 LOCATION

Lerna is located in the southeast corner of the plain of Argos, in southern Greece, on the southern shore of the Bay of Argos (Angel 1971a). The site is adjacent to the modern town of Myloi (Map 16) (Caskey 1954; Caskey & Blackburn 1997). The human skeletal remains are located in the Museum of Argos, Greece.

2.3.2.2 SETTING

The settlement of Lerna has Mount Pontinus behind it, the beach in front of it and two fresh water springs to the north (Map 17) (Angel 1971a; Caskey and Blackburn 1997). There was also access to rich fields to the north and to the south (Caskey 1954). Lerna is nearby the modern city of Nauplion and a close distance from the ancient settlements of Asine and Tiryns. The people of Lerna had easy access to the Cycladic Islands towards the southeast, as well as access through the mountains into Arcadia to the southwest (Angel 1971a).

2.3.2.3 HISTORY

The site was recognised as pre-Mycenaean by A. Frickenhaus and W. Müller in 1909. The first surveys by the American School of Classical Studies were carried out in 1952, which led to seven seasons of excavation from 1952-1958 (Caskey and Blackburn 1997). J. Lawrence Angel studied the human remains in 1954 and 1957 (Angel 1971a).

2.3.2.4 TIME PERIOD

The time period of the site encompasses 7 periods from the Neolithic up to the Late Mycenaean period (Caskey and Blackburn 1997) (Table 2.5). There is also evidence of Geometric, pre-Classical and Hellenistic levels (Caskey 1954). There are some human remains from the Neolithic and Mycenaean periods but only those from the Middle Helladic (Lerna V) were studied.

Lerna Levels	Chronology	Dates
I	Neolithic Early	
II	Neolithic Late	
III	Early Helladic II	2900-2300 BC
IV	Early Helladic III	2300-2100 BC
V	Middle Helladic	2100-1550 BC
VI	Late Helladic I-II	1550-1375 BC
VII	Late Helladic III	1375-1050 BC

Table 2.5 – Chronological sequence of cultural phases at Lerna (Dickinson 1995 pp 19)

2.3.2.5 TYPE OF SITE

The site should be considered a small town with an oval shape and measuring 180 m east to west and 160 m north to south (Caskey and Blackburn 1997). The houses are large and rectangular, sometimes having tiled roofs and protected by heavy fortifications with watchtowers (Angel 1971a). The MH settlement at Lerna seems to have been extensive and prosperous (Caskey and Blackburn 1997). The MH settlement has a long sequence of successive buildings, destruction and rebuilding (Caskey 1955).

2.3.2.6 LOCATION, TYPE AND NUMBER OF TOMBS

The Middle Bronze Age people of Lerna buried their dead under the floors and beside their houses (Caskey 1960; Angel 1971a; Howell 1973). The practice of burying the dead under and among the houses became more frequent during the middle and later phases of the MH, continuing into the LH I period and also to some extent during the Mycenaean period (Caskey 1957). The Middle Bronze Age burials are spread throughout Late Lerna IV (Late Early Helladic III), Lerna V (Middle Helladic), and Lerna VI (Middle Helladic end, and Late Helladic I) (Angel 1971a). The grave types are cist and pit graves, with most of the bodies buried in a contracted position with the head to the north (Caskey 1954; 1958).

Since the people of Lerna buried their dead close to and under their houses, Angel had grouped the burials into 27 family groups and subsequently into 13 clans (Angel 1971a). For this study Angel's breakdown has not been considered. The reason is the number of these groups is too small to conduct accurate bio-distance analysis within the assemblage. The excavated graves yielded a large amount of skeletal remains. Angel suggests the excavators took particular care to collect as many skeletal remains as possible (Angel 1971a). The soil conditions were also favourable for preservation, unlike at Souskiou and Lemba (Cyprus) and at other sites in Greece (Angel 1971a).

2.3.2.7 GRAVE GOODS

Pottery makes up most of the grave goods from the tombs at Lerna. The pottery of the MH has the first appearance of Minyan and Matt-painted wares (Forsén 1992). Another type of pottery is a hard, gritty, handmade ware of light colour, which is very abundant at Lerna V. Fragments, of this type of pottery, have been found at Asine (Frödin & Persson 1938) but seem to be rare or missing at other sites (Caskey 1960). Some other artefacts discovered include sickles of obsidian and flint, grinding slabs and rubbers/pounders (Nordquist, 1987). There is evidence for an increased number of foreign objects found in Lerna V, including the earliest Middle Minoan ceramic styles (Caskey 1960; Rutter 1993).

2.3.3 SUMMARY

The main differences between Lerna and Asine are their size and relative importance in the region. Asine is a small town with an acropolis, with stone built cist, pithoi, shaft and simple earth-cut graves inside and outside the settlement area. Lerna is a small town without being associated with an acropolis where the dead were buried under the floors of the houses and the main grave types are cist and pit graves. The most common type of tomb throughout the MH and at both sites was the earth-cut pit grave, used for children as well as adults and for both sexes. The grave goods found at Asine are very basic but with much variety: some matt-painted pottery, shell, obsidian flakes, arrowheads, fish vertebrae and bones of small animals, bronze tweezers. Pottery makes up most of the grave goods from the tombs at Lerna. Both sites are on the coast with direct access to the sea.

2.4 SYRIA:

The last site, included in this study, is the Early Bronze Age site of Jerablus-Tahtani (hereafter Jerablus) in northern Syria. The Syrian site allows comparison with Cyprus from an eastern perspective. The site of Jerablus is roughly contemporary to the three Chalcolithic sites from Cyprus.

2.4.1 JERABLUS-TAHTANI
2.4.1.1 LOCATION

The site is located in the northwestern part of Syria on the west bank of the Euphrates River approximately 4 km south of Carchemish, Turkey (Map 1) (Peltenburg et al. 1995). The skeletal remains are stored at the University of Edinburgh, the University of Glasgow and at the Lemba Archaeological Centre in Cyprus.

2.4.1.2 SETTING

The site is a Tell and lies on a terrace on the floodplain of the Euphrates river. Since other sites along the river are well back from the flood plain, this puts Jerablus in a unique position. Location on the floodplain has caused the site's eastern side to be eroded slightly (Peltenburg et al. 1995).

2.4.1.3 HISTORY

Sir Leonard Woolley first referred to the site while excavating at Carchemish (Woolley 1921), but did not excavate there, the site was later surveyed by Copeland and Moore (Peltenburg et al. 1995). The recent excavation by the University of Edinburgh under the direction of Peltenburg lasted for six seasons between 1992-2000. This was a rescue excavation in advance of the Tishreen and other dam projects, along the Euphrates River (Peltenburg et al. 1995).

2.4.1.4 TIME PERIOD

The site has a long history from the Late Chalcolithic (Uruk Period) (Period 1), through Early Bronze Age (Period 2), Late Iron Age (Period 3) and Hellenistic to Late Roman (Period 4), to Islamic (Period 5) (Peltenburg et al. 1995:4) (Table 2.6). The human remains come from burials in the Uruk Period (1) and Early Bronze (2) (3rd Millennium). Period 2 has the funerary complex and fortification system (Peltenburg et al. 1995:6). Only the Early Bronze settlement, which is Period 1 and 2, will be considered in this study. Period 2 seemed to be going through a change from a pre-fort to a fortified phase (Peltenburg et al. 1996:5).

JT Periods	Time Period	Dates
Period 1	Late Chalcolithic (Uruk)	3500-3000 BC
Period 2	Early Bronze Age	3000-2400 BC
Period 3	Late Iron Age	5th and 6th Centuries BC
Period 4	Hellenistic to Late Roman	
Period 5	Islamic	

Table 2.6 – Chronological sequence at Jerablus (Modified from Peltenburg et al. 1995:4 and tentative radiocarbon dates from E. Peltenburg pers. comm. 2003).

2.4.1.5 TYPE OF SITE

The site can be considered a small town and may have been in some form of subordinate relationship to the nearby site of Carchemish. Jerablus may also have been an independent trading post (Peltenburg et al. 1995). There is evidence the town was walled and enclosed an area approximately 300 m² (Peltenburg et al. 1996; 1997).

2.4.1.6 LOCATION, TYPE AND NUMBER OF TOMBS

The human remains studied were from the excavations from 1993 to 1998. The site was also excavated in 1999 and 2000, although I was not able to study the remains from those latest two years. Approximately 55 tombs were excavated from 1993 to 1998. The tombs appear to be within the walls of the Period 2 settlement, but the exact location of the wall has not been fully determined (Peltenburg et al. 2000b). There are five types of tombs found at Jerablus:

1. Pithos Burials
2. Shaft Graves
3. Pit Graves
4. Cists
5. Chamber Tombs

A funeral complex in Area II (Period 2) has been identified, comprising the monumental Tomb 302 with satellite burials in pithoi (Map 18) (Peltenburg et al. 1995). This large tomb rivals many other large centres during the Uruk Period, such as Mari and Tell Ahmar in Syria (Peltenburg et al. 1995). Tomb 302 is an above ground tomb with 2 distinct phases. It is a rectangular shaped chamber tomb, with corbelled walls, approximately 6.6 x 3.5 m, oriented east-west with the entrance on the short west side (Peltenburg et al. 1995). Excavation has shown the tomb is also enclosed within a mound. There was no roof identified at the time of this writing, although there is some evidence that a roof may have existed and was possibly removed (Peltenburg et al. 1995).

Burials have also been found under Building 1000, which is rare for the Middle and Upper Euphrates river valley where the normal practice is to bury individuals within cemeteries (Peltenburg et al. 1996).

2.4.1.7 GRAVE GOODS

Tomb 302 has yielded many wealthy objects such as beads, ivory, ostrich egg fragments, gold and imported pottery (Peltenburg et al. 1995). "Access to exotic goods also denotes high standing in society." (Peltenburg et al. 1995:12). In Tomb 302 there was a large concentration of 'Champagne pots', Plain and Simple Ware bowls and corrugated and plain goblets. This assemblage is similar to other sites in the area with similar chamber tombs (Peltenburg et al. 1995). In Tomb 302 a great deal of pottery was deposited over time with some of it broken after deposition due to the multiple periods of disturbance throughout the use of the tomb (Peltenburg et al. 1995).

The other burials have yielded an assortment of pottery as well as copper pins and bracelets. The quality of goods equals those from Tomb 302 as well as from other sites in the area (Peltenburg et al. 1995).

2.4.2 SUMMARY

The main point about Jerablus is that it is a small town on the Euphrates River near the ancient city of Carchemish. This is important because such an important town would influence any smaller communities around it. This may be the reason that, for its size, Jerablus has one of the largest and richest chamber tombs (Tomb 302) of the Uruk Period, such as Mari and Tell Ahmar in Syria. The size and grandness of Tomb 302 is definitely too grand for such a small town. Perhaps the proximity of Jerablus to Carchemish explains the social relationship and possibly the biological relationship in the region. Burials under houses are rare and are found mostly in cemeteries, and in a variety of types such as pithos burials, shaft, pit graves, cists and chamber tombs.

CHAPTER 3

ANTHROPOLOGICAL METHODS

3.1 INTRODUCTION

Standard anthropological data such as age, sex of individuals and stature have been collected for this study. To assess the biological affinities of the different groups, non-metric data from the teeth and cranial and post-cranial skeleton have also been collected. Each type of data will be explained in the following pages.

3.2 STATE OF PRESERVATION

Before the different data collection methods are explained, a word must be said on the state of preservation of the various human remains that were studied. The state of preservation ranged from extremely poor (for example from the site of Souskiou) to excellent (from the site of Lerna). The condition of the remains depended on three factors: the initial soil and grave conditions, the excavation and retrieval methods utilised by the excavators, and conditions in which the human remains were stored in the various museums and storage rooms. This is important when considering some of the remains studied were excavated as long as 75 years ago. When dealing with such old remains, extra attention was given to the reports from the anthropologists who studied them at the time of excavation. Their initial observations are invaluable and greatly enhanced this study. In some instances, where my interpretations of some aspect of the identification of the remains differed, the original observer's interpretation was used. Even though there have been many advances in the study of human remains through the years, it is important to recognise the remains may have been damaged during their decades in storage and their altered appearance could affect the interpretation.

The degree of skeletal completeness for each of the samples varied. In the earlier part of the century, because of the focus on metrical study of the cranium, mostly crania were retained from excavations, and perhaps the occasional long bone such as the femur. Such was the case from the Swedish Expedition to Cyprus during the 1920's. This automatically limits the information that can be extracted from the incomplete remains. The Swedish Expedition to Greece was a little more thorough with their collecting of human remains, but there appeared to be a lack of teeth from the remains. Out of approximately 145 individuals from the site of Asine, approximately 154 teeth were identified. This greatly affects the outcome of the dental non-metric analysis as well as the age determination.

3.3 MINIMUM NUMBER OF INDIVIDUALS (MNI)

The minimum number of individuals (hereafter MNI) of each sample needed to be determined before any analysis could begin. Although sounding straightforward this procedure is often complicated and some of the sites studied proved interesting challenges in determining the MNI.

To estimate MNI, the information on which bones were present had to be determined. This was accomplished by traveling to the various locations where the collections were stored and producing a catalogue of all human bones present. All of the human remains used in this study came from inhumations, the tomb structures ranging from simple pit graves to elaborate mortuary structures. The number of inhumations from each tomb also varied from a single interment to over one dozen. The standard practice when recording human physical remains is to examine all the remains in a grave and then determine how many individuals are present and the age, sex and so on of each. The nature of the skeletal remains and how they were stored dictated a different method for determining the MNI to be developed. In some cases, human remains from multiple burial tombs had been stored collectively in the same bag. Therefore, many individuals were present in one bag, which meant each bone needed to be treated as a separate individual. The age and sex were therefore determined for each bone (some individual bones cannot be aged or sexed adequately or at all). Only when all of the bags were checked could the bones be sorted by age and sex, using Microsoft Access™. At this point it was determined how many individuals were present and to which age group they belonged (the age and sex methods I utilised will be discussed later). Many extra notes were taken to assist in determining the MNI, such as size and morphology of each bone and any unusual features of the bones.

The Syrian site of Jerablus had a unique mortuary structure - Tomb 302. This tomb posed many difficulties in analysis and interpretation for the excavation team (which is presently working on a comprehensive publication for the site). Tomb 302 is a large stone built tomb approximately 6.6 x 3.5 m by 2m in height. The meticulous excavation and recording methods utilised by the archaeologists greatly assisted the analysis of the individuals found within the tomb. Many of the bones excavated from the tomb were assigned numbers, which were then marked on the plan of each level excavated. None of the individuals in the tomb was found in anatomical position, therefore the bone numbers were used in concert with their location on the tomb plan, along with the age and sex information about each bone. Through a slow process, individuals of similar age and sex for the entire tomb were matched up. There is no easy method in determining MNI, which is fraught with difficulties on such a complicated tomb, but I believe the method used, combining bone age, sex and morphology along with bone number and stratigraphic sequence, minimised any errors.

3.4 AGE ESTIMATION

As mentioned above, individual bones were identified from graves and the age and sex of each bone was determined for a single tomb. Only when all of the remains from a single tomb had been recorded could an accurate identification of age and sex be determined. This method proved to be very useful when dealing with graves with an unknown number of individuals. By comparing all of the age estimates from the different methods, e.g. teeth, cranial sutures, bone fusion and others, the specific age or even age range for an individual was determined. The age estimates from the different methods usually agreed with one another and when some age estimates fell outside the range of expected values were discarded when examining the whole.

3.4.1 AGE ESTIMATION METHODS

Even though all of the assemblages except for Jerablus were previously published, the age of each individual was determined. For some remains, obviously damaged through years in storage, the age the anthropologist who previously studied them was accepted over the author's estimate. J.L. Angel (1971) previously studied the human remains from Lerna, and on the whole our age estimation of adults was in agreement. Angel's age estimations of children and infants were ignored, because there have been many advances in the age estimation of children and newer techniques were used.

Varieties of methods were used to determine the age of the large number of remains examined. Because the majority of skeletal remains were those of children, the method used most was tooth formation and eruption (Moorrees et al. 1963a, 1963b; Ubelaker 1989; Smith 1991) as well as long bone length (Hoffman 1979; Scheuer et al. 1980; Hoppa 1992). In some assemblages, a number of foetuses were found and for these bone measurements were used to determine age (Kósa 1989).

Determining the age at death of adults and sub-adults is different from that of children. For sub-adults, the most used methods are tooth development and eruption, long bone length and epiphyseal fusion of long bones and other bones (Bass 1987; Schwartz 1995). In many instances an individual, still in the developmental stage, had one skeletal element fully mature while another element was not, which forces the anthropologist to place individuals within an age range rather than assign a definite age. Another factor to consider is each population may reach maturity at a different age. The tables and data sets used by anthropologists are mostly from people who lived in the 19th and 20th centuries (usually from Europe and North America) may have had different maturity rates from prehistoric peoples (Lunt 1994).

Methods used for determining the age at death of adults and mature adults were the examination of tooth wear (Lovejoy 1985), pubic symphysis stages (Gilbert & McKern 1973; Katz & Suchey 1986), cranial suture closure (Meindl & Lovejoy 1985), age-related changes in the proximal epiphysis of the humerus and femur (Acsadi & Nemeskeri 1970) and occasionally, even age estimation from rib ends (Işcan et al. 1984a, 1984b, 1985).

Given the inherent problems with incomplete skeletal assemblages, many age techniques as possible were used in determining the age of individuals. Many age techniques examine age related degenerative effects on the skeleton (e.g. dental wear and cranial suture closure), and these become more inaccurate the older the individual becomes (Hershkovitz et al. 1997). Caution should always be used when too little of the skeleton is present for a proper age assessment.

3.4.2 AGE GROUPS

The age groups used in this study were divided into seven stages (Table 3.1). First is the Infant stage, from birth to eleven months of life; any foetuses found have also been included in this stage. The second stage is Child 1, from older than one year to six years old. The next stage is Child 2, from 7 to 12 years, which is the end of childhood, just before the processes of maturation begin.

The next stage is Sub-Adult (adolescent) where the long bones go through their last growing phase, almost all of the teeth have erupted and the bones begin to show signs of sexual dimorphism (Ubelaker 1989; Smith 1991). When determining age, one of the most difficult stages determined is between the Sub-Adult and Adult 1 groups. Adult 1 is the stage for final tooth eruption, specifically of the third molar (Smith 1991), final fusion of many bones (Schwartz 1995), changes in the pelvis (Gilbert & McKern 1973; Katz & Suchey 1986) and rib ends (Işcan et al. 1984a, 1984b, 1985). The assessing of age from dental wear after the teeth have fully erupted can begin at this stage (Lovejoy 1985). Dental wear can be affected by the amount of abrasive material in the diet, along with the amount of wear on the dentition caused by other activities such as gripping with the teeth.

Adult 2 represents, in skeletal maturation terms, middle age and can be determined from assessing the stage of cranial suture fusion (Meindl & Lovejoy 1985). Dental wear and pubic symphysis changes are also useful criteria to determine age at this stage. Adult 3 stage represents the mature period, when all the cranial bones have fused or are in the process of fusing. Dental wear is usually extreme by this last stage, making it difficult to accurately estimate age. Usually a heavily worn dentition would classify as extreme age. As mentioned above regarding tooth wear, by this age in pre-industrial societies most teeth are heavily worn and an advanced age can be assumed, but such an age should be supported with other age indicators. After the mid-forties to 50, age cannot be accurately determined, so the Adult 3 range is 46+.

Since many ageing methods were used to determining the age of individuals, in most cases an age range was the result for an individual. Therefore, the mean age was selected from all the methods used.

Age groups	Age ranges
Infant	(0-11 mo)
Child 1	(>1-6)
Child 2	(7-12)
Sub Adult	(13-18)
Adult 1	(19-30)
Adult 2	(31-45)
Adult 3	(46+)

Table 3.1 – Age groups

3.5 SEX DETERMINATION

Remains studied which were in poorer condition than when first excavated, the sex determination by the anthropologist who studied them previously was invaluable. A standard practice by today's physical anthropologists is not to assign sex to any individual younger than adult age. Some of the previously published reports from the assemblage have assigned sex to children as young as 1 year old. It should be noted the purpose here is not to undermine the anthropologist's skill and expertise, which some have developed for decades. What my experience has taught me about the development of the skeleton is determining the sex of an individual before the years of adulthood is very difficult and becomes less reliable the younger the individual is. It is the belief of this anthropologist the earliest one can confidently sex an individual is late adolescence, and age may be different for each cultural group. It is more reliable to determine the sex of adults from 19 years and older.

Sex was assigned to adults and older sub-adults, and was determined by examining the traits on the skull, pelvis and measurements from some of the long bones (Dittrick & Suchey 1986). On the skull, features observed were the nuchal ridge, temporal lines, height, slope and shape of frontal and the shape of parietals (Keen 1950; Schwartz 1995). On the mandible, thickness of mandibular body, flaring of gonial angles, and ramus angle; on the pelvis, sciatic notch, pubic symphysis, pubic angle, overall shape of pelvis, sacrum and supra-auricular sulcus (Washburn 1948; Phenice 1969; Krogman & Işcan 1986; Sutherland & Suchey 1991).

Measurements from adult long bones also assisted in determining sex of many individuals, especially when no fragments of the pelvis or cranium were present. Width measurement of the humeral and femoral heads along with distal and proximal radii were taken and compared to tables to determine whether they fell into the male or female range. These tables are based on measurements from modern populations of known sex and body type (Bass 1987).

When using these methods to identify sex, some assumptions are required for the conclusions to be accepted. The main assumption is there will be an observable degree of sexual dimorphism between males and females. This means males are generally larger and more robust than females, and this can be identified on the skeletal frame. The long bone measurements and some of the traits from the skull and mandible are dependant on the robustness of each person, which can be affected by the degree of physical labour the individual was subject to in life as well as the level of nutrition during the formation of the bones in childhood and in later life. Skeletal diseases can also affect bone growth and thickness. Finally, the degree of sexual dimorphism may be slightly different between populations, while sexed individuals are assumed 'normal' for that population.

The state of preservation as well as the burial practices of the assemblages dictated which sexing methods were used. For example, the well-preserved and well-stored collection from Lerna allowed for using sexing methods for the pelvis, cranium and long bone epiphyseal measurements (Angel's publication (1971) on the assemblage allowed for corroboration of the sexing). In contrast, the assemblage from Souskiou, which has much worse preservation and storage allowed mostly cranial sexing methods.

3.6 DEMOGRAPHY

The age data determined from the remains will be used to reconstruct demographic profiles for each sample. These life tables display the structure and dynamics of the population by combining all of the individuals in the sample, so the community can be examined as a single unit. The data can then quickly and efficiently compared to other samples, modern or ancient. The basis of the life tables for ancient populations is the age estimation determined by the anthropologist, therefore the results from the life tables are only as good as the methods used to age the individuals (Angel 1969; Chamberlain 2000; Gage 2000). This must always be kept in mind when studying ancient populations.

Resulting from the difficulties inherent in the age assessment of ancient populations, anthropologists continue to question and improve on current methods. Life tables need to be developed which more accurately represent ancient and more diverse populations than tables currently available. This researcher is well aware of the limitations of the data collection and the interpretation methods available. For information about the critiques on demography, please refer to Milner (et al. 1989) and Konigsberg and Frankenberg (1992).

3.7 STATURE

For stature estimation, length of the adult upper and lower limb bones were measures and compared to various stature tables (Trotter & Gleser 1952; Trotter 1970). The main stature table used was based on known long bone lengths and stature of modern white males and females from the United States. By using this source, certain assumptions must be made and considered for these results to have any meaning. First, the data in the tables are overall considered to be from people who have had the benefit of a modern western medical system and had possibly not been subject to malnutrition as children. These two basic assumptions can greatly affect the stature estimates of the ancient people under consideration. One method of achieving a more accurate estimate of stature is to measure the height of the entire skeleton, from the foot bones, through the lower limbs and the entire vertebral column, to the cranium. Unfortunately, the majority of the skeletal remains studied were far too incomplete for such calculations to be made.

Some of the long bones studied were incomplete so partial measurements were taken and applied to a regression formula (Steele & McKern 1969; Steele 1970) specifically designed to determine the stature of the individual from fragmentary bone. Again, part of the problem with the regression formula is it is based on modern western people (mostly Europeans), which may have little of no bearing on ancient people from the eastern Mediterranean (Feldesman & Fountain 1996). Stature information gained from this study should be used merely as a guide and for comparison with other studies, which use the popular Trotter and Steele methods.

3.8 NON-METRIC TRAITS
3.8.1 INTRODUCTION

Along with the anthropological data in this study, the collection and analysis of non-metric traits will also be used to determine the biological affinities of the different populations. The history of non-metric traits has been well documented in other studies and the purpose of this discussion is not to go over the history again (Berry & Berry 1967; Ossenberg 1976; Saunders 1978; Scott & Turner 1997; Tyrrell 2000). The nature and scope of this study will allow an explanation of the traits used and some of the arguments for their uses and their limitations will be discussed here.

Non-metric traits "are minor variants of phenotypic expression" (Tyrrell 2000: 290). They can be present in all human tissue but those present in bone and teeth are most suited for anthropologists. Non-metric traits have been used in other studies to compare the biological affinities of different populations (Anderson 1968; De Villiers 1968; Berry & Berry 1972; Rightmire 1972: Sofaer et al. 1972; Finnegan 1974; Corruccini 1974; C. Berry 1976; Carpenter 1976; Ossenberg 1976; Saunders 1978; Turner & Swindler 1978; Turner 1979; Dutta 1984; Lukacs & Walimbe 1984; Sjøvold 1984; Turner & Markowitz 1990; Irish & Turner 1990; Hemphill et al. 1991; Lukacs & Hemphill 1991; Johnson & Lovell 1994; Alt et al. 1997; Scott & Turner 1997; Coppa et al. 1998; Irish 1998; Cucina et al. 1999; Irish 2000). Non-metric traits are also referred to as quasi-continuous traits (Grünberg 1952). Grünberg used that term because the traits were not controlled by simple Mendelian genetics, but are also affected by environmental factors (Hiernaux 1963; Tyrrell 2000).

Most of these traits occur as a variation in the bone or dental characteristics in all humans (these traits also occur in other mammals). These variations can be as simple as a pit, groove or facet on the bone surface or as complex as extra cusps and roots in the dentition. In cranial and post-cranial bones, non-metric traits can be scored as either present or absent, while in dentition the degree of expression is also graded. None of the samples considered here had previously been examined for non-metric traits. These traits are collected by a simple visual inspection of the particular skeletal element. The recording of these traits does not require any special tools but does require training in identification.

This study will compare samples by using a combination of traits, not single traits. Previous studies on cranial metrics, as well as cranial morphology, treated individuals as representatives of a population. In this study, the unit of comparison will be the entire sample. The dynamics of the gene pool encompass the entire population and not just the extremes.

3.8.2 SIDE CONSIDERATIONS

The way the traits are counted directly affects the accuracy of statistical analysis. The incidence of traits can be calculated by individual (Tyrrell 2000) or by side of body (Berry & Berry 1967; Berry 1975; Tyrrell 2000). Because the skeletal samples were often in poor condition, the approach of counting all bones individually and hence each trait individually was used. One drawback of this method is bilateral traits are counted twice increasing the amount of information collected (Saunders 1978; Ossenberg 1981 Nichol 1989). Each method has its drawbacks but with small samples, as in this study, have it is acceptable to count all the traits (Scott and Turner 1997; Irish 2000; Tyrrell 2000).

There is still disagreement between scholars regarding the problem of recording by side or by individual. Saunders points out that recording by side introduces redundancy to the calculating of the distance statistic (Saunders 1978). Recording by side does not greatly affect one way or the other the measure of divergence and does not find significant side differences for trait frequencies when total side occurrences (including bilateral occurrences) are compared (Saunders 1978; Ossenberg 1981). Saunders states significance testing on the left and right sides has shown "...the degree of significant differences in side incidence were found to be low and therefore it was felt sides could be justifiably pooled" (Saunders 1978:28-29). It is also important to remember asymmetries, which do occur for some traits, may not be simply random but related to basic physiological asymmetries (Saunders 1978; Trinkaus 1978). Most of these studies relate to non-dental skeletal traits, which behave differently from teeth. Teeth usually (but not always) exhibit left-right symmetry (Garn 1966; Scott & Turner 1997: 96).

3.8.3 SEX CONSIDERATIONS

The small samples did not allow this study to consider the differences between sexes, in regards to the analysis of non-metric traits. By separating each sample by sex, the already small number of individuals becomes even smaller creating more uncertainty with the statistical analysis. Even though the assemblage from Lerna was large, the smaller commingled tombs from Souskiou and Jerablus did not permit for dividing male and female dentition. A uniform method was used for all sites. Therefore, sexes were not subjected to the χ^2 significance test. A larger sample of human remains, at least 100 of each sex, would be a better basis to consider the distribution of non-metric traits among sexes. Berry and Berry (1967) consider the differences between sex in trait frequencies not significantly different, so male and female can be combined (Turner et al. 1991; Hanihara 1992; Irish 1997; Irish 2000). Bang and Hasund also found there was no sex difference for shovel shaped incisors and the Carabelli trait (Bang and Hasund 1971; 1972). Conversely, Corruccini (1974) argues that separating samples by sex is imperative to understand the biological dynamics of the population. Anderson (1968) had also noticed trait differences by sex in his studies. A number of studies on cranial traits have tested the significance of differences between males and females and concluded there are some significant differences (Saunders 1978). The traits should be separated by sex when possible but, if this is not possible, the differences are not very great and do not substantially affect the results (Anderson 1968; Corruccini 1974; Saunders 1978). Grünberg suggests sex differences in trait frequency may generally reflect size differences as expressions of sexual dimorphism (Grünberg 1952). Observed differences between the sexes should be tested by χ^2 for significance (Tyrrell 2000).

Although the samples were not separated by sex, a breakdown of sites by sex was prepared to show the sex ratio for all sites. The table shows at every site, except Lemba, there are more males than females (Tale 3.2). Although the breakdown between the sites is not consistent, the percentage of males ranges from 10.3% (AS) to 64.3% (EN). The percentage of adults of unknown sex is as high and even higher than many of the sexed adults. This table helps to illustrate the small sample of sexed individuals and high number of unsexed individuals of most of the sites that did not allow for a breakdown by sex for this study.

	LL		SOU		KM		AI		EN		AS		LER		JT	
	No.	%	No.	%	No.	%	No.	%	No.	%	No.	%	No.	%	No.	%
SA	5	25	6	22.2	5.5	17.7	3	7.14	1	1.43	4	10.3	8	7.9	4	8.9
M	5	25	5	18.5	11	35.5	27	64.3	34	48.6	4	10.3	51	50.5	15	33.3
F	8	40	3	11.1	13	41.9	12	28.6	24	34.3	2	5.1	40	39.6	13	28.9
UK	2	10	13	48.1	1.5	4.84	0	0	11	15.7	29	74.4	2	1.98	13	28.9
	20	100	27	100	31	100	42	100	70	100	39	100	101	100	45	100

Table 3.2 – Breakdown by sex of all sub-adults and adults from all sites

3.8.4 AGE DIFFERENCES

Age is also a factor with the formation and development of non-metric traits and will be discussed separately with each of the different types of non-metric traits collected. This study observed traits from the dentition and cranial and post-cranial skeletons.

3.8.5 DENTAL NON-METRIC TRAITS

State of preservation was an important factor with this series of remains, so the main source of non-metric data comes from teeth. This study looked at thirty-five dental traits, found in people around the world, from the list prepared by the Arizona State University (ASU) (Turner et al. 1991). This list and variations of it have been used in other non-metric studies (Lee & Goose 1972; Berry 1978; Turner &

Swindler 1978; Turner 1979; Turner 1987; Irish & Turner 1990; Turner & Markowitz 1990; Hemphill et al. 1991; Johnson & Lovell 1994; Irish 1995; 1997; Stringer et al. 1997; Irish 1998; Irish 2000).

The ASU list of dental traits is also accompanied by a set of plaster casts, which display each trait with a series of teeth from an absence of the trait to strong presence. Much time was spent studying the ASU plaster casts in the lab at the University of Sheffield. The casts were not available to take into the field when examining the various dental collections, but this did not pose a great problem in analysis and interpretation because of the way the data was selected for the statistical analysis. The traits ultimately included in the statistical analysis were those, which showed a definite presence, not merely a faint presence. Therefore, this selection process has nullified whatever errors may be present from any inconsistency in recording the dental traits.

An acceptable level of proficiency was developed in identifying the various traits and the degree of expression of each trait. In the end, over 3,500 teeth were examined making the traits easier to identify and record. Assistance was also received from Drs. Andrew Chamberlain and Dorothy Lunt on the identification of the traits.

The dental traits were recorded from the permanent dentition. Since the permanent teeth form in children at a very young age, it was possible to include individuals from as young as 1 year old. This was a great advantage for two reasons: first, more of the population was included in this study, and second, given the high infant mortality rate in prehistoric populations, there was a high proportion of young unworn teeth to examine for traits. Another advantage is teeth are very durable and even in very young individuals survive better than fragile bones (Bang & Hasund 1971; Berry 1976). The disadvantages with dental traits are extreme age usually obliterates traits in mature adults, and large amounts of abrasive material in the diet may create difficulties when traits are too worn to be recorded accurately. Since the majority of adults come from the middle age groups (19-30 & 31-45) and not the oldest age group (46+), this suggests that the exclusion of the elderly from the non-metric analysis due to heavily worn teeth accounts for a small part of the population. Therefore, it is not suspected to greatly affect the outcome of the analysis.

Non-metric traits from teeth have been used mainly in comparing the relationship between skeletal samples and are not well suited for comparing relatedness between different individuals (Tyrrell 2000). Some examples of this are the long-standing work by Christy G. Turner II and colleagues over the last three decades. Turner and colleagues have used dental traits to understand migration in East and South East Asia (Turner 1976; Turner & Swindler 1978; Turner 1979; Scott 1980; Turner 1987; Turner & Markowitz 1990; Scott & Turner 1997). Dental traits have also been used to compare the biological affinities of the people of modern Europe with Neanderthals (Stringer et al. 1997; Tyrrell & Chamberlain 1998). The conclusions from both of these studies suggest Neanderthals are significantly distinct from modern humans suggesting *Homo sapiens sapiens* did indeed replace Neanderthals in Europe. This conclusion has also been supported by a study using modern DNA from Europe and the Middle East (Richards et al. 1996). Although traits from all around the body will be recorded, only dental traits will be used in the analysis of biological affinities. This is mainly because according to Turner: "Teeth are well known for their evolutionary conservatism and high genetic component in their occurrence." (1976:912). This makes them effective in the analysis of the different populations.

3.8.6 CRANIAL NON-METRIC TRAITS

As well as dental traits, non-metric traits from the cranium and the mandible were recorded. A cranial traits list prepared by Berry & Berry (1967) was adopted which lists and describes thirty non-metric cranial traits. Before Berry and Berry published their landmark paper on the use of cranial traits, anthropologists primarily conducted distance studies using cranial metrics. Berry and Berry suggested, as well as being suitable for distance studies, non-metric traits had the added advantage of being useful even when the bones were fragmentary (Berry & Berry 1967). Obviously with cranial metrics, a damaged or incomplete skull made measurement more difficult. There have since been many distance studies using cranial traits (Nielsen 1970; Nielsen 1972; Carpenter 1976; Ossenberg 1976; Green et al. 1979; Molto 1979; Sciulli 1990).

Age is an important factor with cranial traits. Ossenberg (1970) suggests the differences between adults and juveniles are small and, assuming the proportions are equal, consider it acceptable to allow for pooling of traits from the two age groups. Other researchers disagree with Ossenberg, suggesting traits should be recorded for each age group (juveniles and adults) and compared separately because the traits are expressed differently through age (Corruccini, 1974). Nevertheless, due to the small samples in this study, in order not to divide the samples even further all adult traits were combined. As mentioned earlier, only traits from individuals over 18 years of age were included in the sample of the adults.

Berry and Berry (1967) did not test their sample for age related differences, while Ossenberg (1970) and Buikstra (1972) both found that age did affect the trait frequency. Buikstra (1972) even suggests individuals below the age of 12 should be dropped from a sample altogether. Berry (1975) suggested if the sample is mainly adult material, then age is not as much of a factor. This present study only included cranial non-metric traits from individuals over the age of 18.

Some cranial traits have been known to be affected by artificial head deformation practiced by many peoples around the world (Bennett 1965). Accessory sutural bones, which can be found in the lambdoidal suture, have been known to appear in higher than normal frequencies when cranial deformation is present (Ossenberg 1970; Gottlieb 1978).

3.8.7 POST-CRANIAL NON-METRIC TRAITS

Along with the dentition and cranium, traits from the post-cranial skeleton were collected using a list prepared by Finnegan (1978), which documents thirty non-metric post-cranial traits (also called infra-cranial traits). Finnegan (1978) suggested post-cranial traits would be better suited for distance studies because:

1. All traits considered have the possibility of bilateral expression
2. Most of the traits are found on heavy bone materials which are most apt to survive prolonged burial and subsequent excavation
3. Many of these traits have a long history of studies dealing with sex and side dimorphism.

There have been many studies on post-cranial traits (Finnegan 1974; Finnegan & Cooprinder 1978; Saunders 1978; Saunders & Popovich 1978; Conner 1990). From his studies on side differences, Finnegan (1978) determined there was no significant difference. Finnegan (1978) suggests a similar study done on the same sample but with cranial traits did show some significant differences by side. Finnegan (1978) also noted fewer differences, with post-cranial traits, when it came to the differences between the sexes, unlike the differences between the sexes with the cranial traits. As with the cranial traits, only traits from skeletally mature individuals were used in this study.

3.8.8 PROBLEMS WITH TRAIT COLLECTION

Aside from the specific considerations of each set of traits, inter-observer error is the most important factor to consider with all of the traits (Corruccini 1974; Molto 1979). With regard to inter-observer error Scott and Turner state:

> "We grant there are problems in this area but also maintain that the problems have been overstated, they are not insurmountable, and their order of magnitude is no greater than that involved in blood typing where scales of agglutination are used." (Scott & Turner 1997:70).

Scott and Dahlberg (1982) suggest inter-observer error accounts for between 5-10% of the variation in a study. Therefore, such errors, which may have occurred in this study, have not greatly affected the results. Standardisation has also been a major concern to anthropologists using non-metric traits to study population distance in terms of which traits to collect, how to define a present trait, and which traits are good genetic indicators. The work by Berry & Berry, Finnegan, Turner and Scott has set some standards for anthropologists to follow. Another factor is the influence from the environment on the traits (Grünberg 1952; Hiernaux 1963; Ossenberg 1972; Saunders 1978; Trinkaus 1978).

3.9 DATA FROM PUBLICATIONS

The anthropological data will also be accompanied by cultural data from the excavations to assist in creating a more accurate picture of the human lifestyles and how they relate to each other and to the period, from which they belong. The main aspect of this study is to compare the biological affinities of the people involved and this can be done by understanding not only their biological affinities through their non-metric traits, but also their lifestyles. One of the main issues when using non-metric traits is the way they are affected by environmental factors. The environmental factors affecting these traits are diet, geographic location and social structure. Social structure is not a natural environmental factor but it does influence people's diet, subsistence pattern, isolation and reproductive habits, which are all factors affecting population dynamics and biological affinities.

3.10 OTHER SOURCES OF GENETIC DATA

When deciding on what type of data to collect for this study, cranial metric data and ancient DNA were also considered to determine the biological affinities of the samples. A considerable amount of time was spent researching the feasibility and possibility of collecting ancient DNA from the human remains in this study. Ancient DNA can be extracted from soft tissue, teeth and bone and even from cremated bone (Brown et al. 1995; Evison et al. 1997; Stone 2000).

A number of problems appeared regarding the possible examination of ancient DNA in this study. The first problem encountered was, all of the sites except for Jerablus are old excavations, begun up to 75 years ago. This crucial factor immediately brings up the question of contamination through excavation, processing and storage (Brown & Brown 1992). The forms of burial rite or inhumation procedure were also sometimes unknown, making it difficult for the researcher to assess whether any ancient DNA came from the individual under study (Brown & Brown 1992). Contamination can also come from other individuals who may have been interred together in an ossuary or communal tomb (Brown & Brown 1992). There are methods available to screen out some of the possible contamination. First, screening out of DNA from people who were exposed to the remains can minimise any recent contamination (Brown & Brown 1992). Clean sterile conditions during excavation are an essential starting point

(Colson et al. 1997). Surface contamination can be removed by grinding away the exposed layers or by soaking the material in hydrochloric acid or a bleach solution (Stone 2000).

For some of the remains it is impossible to screen out any extra DNA from people who have been in contact with the remains (Brown & Brown 1992; Brown et al. 1995; Stone 2000), making the reliability of the DNA extracted questionable. Another reason for rejecting DNA sampling is preservation (Stone 2000). The skeletal remains from Souskiou, for example, have lost much of their collagen; it is mostly mineral which remains in the bones, and the same is true for the dentition, in which only the enamel shell remains from the crowns (Lunt 1985; 1994).

When contamination is not a factor, the type of DNA, which is preferred from human remains, is mitochondrial DNA (mtDNA), which is maternally inherited (Richards et al. 1993; Colson et al. 1997; Stone 2000). MtDNA is easier to recover and is more likely to survive than nuclear DNA (Richards et al. 1993; Stone 2000). It can be used to determine migration, sex or ancestral lineage, but a drawback is by only examining the maternal relations, half of the population is ignored (Brown & Brown 1994; Richards et al. 1996; Stone 2000).

A final factor in rejecting DNA analysis, as a method was cost. It was decided for the scope and time limit of this study that recording the non-metric traits from the bones and teeth would allow for data to be collected in larger quantities and at less cost in time and money than DNA extraction would. In time, it may be possible for DNA extraction techniques to improve and for the specter of contamination to diminish. Until which time when such methods could be used on older skeletal assemblages, the recording of non-metric traits may fill this need for determining the biological affinities of ancient populations.

3.11 CRANIAL METRICS

The methods used in this study have been partly determined by the state of preservation of the human remains. Collecting cranial metrics was also considered, but when the first samples were being studied, it was quickly realised there were no complete crania to measure. As the collections increased in size, some partial and complete crania appeared, but seemed too few to conduct a proper cranial metric study.

CHAPTER 4

DEMOGRAPHY

4.1 INTRODUCTION

For the purpose of this study the sites will be compared first locally then on a greater regional scale. A table combining all of the demographic data and breakdown by sex for all sites is presented for completeness (Table 4.1). Most of the data in this table will be presented again within each regional comparison and where is it not it will be referred to. Since the main focus of this study is southwest Cyprus, these sites will be examined first. As these sites are among the oldest in this study, they also have the added advantage of being in close proximity to each other, creating a large enough sample for comparative studies of other regions. The sites in southwest Cyprus are Souskiou, Lemba-Lakkous and Kissonerga-Mosphilia.

4.2 SOUTHWEST CYPRUS
4.2.1 SOUSKIOU

The skeletal remains studied are from fourteen rock cut tombs. Dr. Dorothy Lunt conducted a study on the human remains, but as they are of such poor quality, she focused primarily on dentition (Lunt 1994). Therefore, this will be the first anthropological report on this site. The MNI for this sample is estimated to be at least 38 individuals (Dr. Lunt recorded 37 individuals). These tombs have been subjected to looting over a long period (as recent as the 1970's), leaving the human as well as the archaeological remains in a very poor state of preservation (Maier & Wartburg 1994). The poor condition of the human bones and teeth is the result of what appears to be a state of semi-fossilization (Lunt 1994). According to Lunt: "The bone appears to have received an influx of calcium salts and is partially petrified." (Lunt 1994: 120). The bones and teeth are very brittle and fragile due to the loss of much of the organic collagen, leaving mostly bone mineral, hindering analysis. Analysis also proved difficult due to the heavily worn condition of the teeth.

Not all of the skeletal material excavated was available for inclusion in this study, so there may be gaps in the data for some or all of the age groups. However, as this study represents a sample of the entire population, it should still be representative of the population as a whole.

	Cyprus										Greece				Syria	
	SOU		KM		LL		AI		EN		AS		LER		JT	
Age Class	D_x	%	D_x	%	D_x	%	D_x	%	D_x	%	D_x	%	D_x	%	D_x	%
I(0-11 mo)	3	7.9	16	20.5	6	11.5	0	0.0	0	0.0	79	54.5	82	35.8	49	39.8
C1(1-6)	3.5	9.2	26.5	34.0	23	44.2	0	0.0	7	8.8	21	14.5	39	17.0	23	18.7
C2(7-12)	0.5	1.3	4.5	5.8	3	5.8	3	6.7	3	3.8	6	4.1	7	3.1	6	4.9
SA(13-18)	6	15.7	5.5	7.1	5	9.6	3	6.7	1	1.3	4	2.8	8	3.5	4	3.3
A1(19-30)M	3	7.9	4	5.1	2	3.8	4	8.9	4	5.0	0	0.0	12	5.2	9	7.3
A1(19-30)F	3	7.9	5	6.4	5	9.6	5	11.1	7	8.8	1	0.7	21	9.2	4	3.3
A1(19-30)UK	10.7	28.1	1.8	2.3	0	0.0	0.6	1.3	4.5	5.6	20	13.8	1.1	0.5	8	6.5
A2(31-45)M	0	0.0	4	5.1	2	3.8	10	22.2	23	28.8	2	1.4	32	14.0	3	2.4
A2(31-45)F	0	0.0	5	6.4	3	5.8	3	6.7	13	16.3	0	0.0	16	7.0	7	5.7
A2(31-45)UK	6	15.7	0.8	1.0	2	3.8	9.6	21.3	1.8	2.3	12	8.3	2.6	1.1	2.9	2.4
A3(46+)M	2	5.2	1	1.3	1	1.9	2	4.4	6	7.5	0	0.0	7	3.1	2	1.6
A3(46+)F	0	0.0	2	2.6	0	0.0	2	4.4	2	2.5	0	0.0	1	0.4	2	1.6
A3(46+)UK	0.4	1.0	1.8	2.3		0.0	2.8	6.2	7.7	9.6	0	0.0	0.3	0.1	3.1	2.5
	38	100	78	100	52	100	45	100	80	100	145	100	229	100	123	100

Table 4.1 – Combined demography and male-female breakdown of all sites (D_x = number of deaths, M = male, F = female and UK = unknown sex).

4.2.2 LEMBA-LAKKOUS

The skeletal remains studied from Lemba-Lakkous (here after Lemba) were from a total of 53 tombs, representing all of the tombs uncovered during the excavation period 1976-1983 (Peltenburg 1985). The MNI from these tombs is 52, with one tomb not yielding any human remains. Dr. Dorothy Lunt completed the anthropological report on the remains, but focused mainly on the dentition (Lunt 1985), whereas this study is concerned with all aspects of the skeleton. According to Lunt:

> "The teeth, usually much better preserved than the bones, were also in rather poor condition. Many had suffered from a kind of *post mortem* erosion in which the surface enamel became chalky and pitted, and a noticeable loss of substance had sometimes occurred." (Lunt 1985:54).

Some teeth were in better condition because they were still protected in the alveolus of the maxilla or mandible (Lunt 1985). In most instances Lunt's age estimates were in agreement with my own. When they were not, I used either Dr. Lunt's estimation or my own, depending on the specific circumstances of each set of remains.

As with many anthropological estimates, the age estimates derived from the teeth were based on the assumption in which the pattern and rates of tooth development in prehistoric Cypriots were similar to modern populations and each child was normal or 'average' (Lunt 1985). According to Dr. Lunt, there is some dispute whether it is reasonable to assume there is no change in the developmental stages of teeth. Some people living in more 'primitive' conditions do experience an earlier eruption stage, such as some African Negro populations (Lunt 1985). Any changes in bone and tooth development must be based on health and nutrition differences rather than on changes in human evolution in the past 6000 years. Age estimation tables are compiled from a specific modern population, so data should be used as a guide only and not as an absolute when comparing populations, which are different in geography or time. While determining the ages for the children from Lemba, Lunt discovered in many cases differences in tooth stage formation occurred within the same set of dentition. This is not uncommon but a high occurrence was observed in the Lemba remains (Lunt 1985).

4.2.3 KISSONERGA-MOSPHILIA

The skeletal remains studied were from a total of 65 tombs. Drs. Dorothy Lunt and Marie Watt studied the dental remains (Lunt et al, 1998). As with the Lemba remains, I compared my results with those of Drs. Lunt and Watt and where there was disagreement, depending on the available remains I choose Dr. Lunt's age estimation or my own. The MNI for this sample is 78 individuals.

4.2.4 SOUTHWEST CYPRIOT DEMOGRAPHY

These three sites are situated in southwest Cyprus in the Paphos District (Map 2). Lemba and Mosphilia are north of Paphos, approximately 1.5 km from each other. Souskiou is east of Paphos, approximately 20 km away from Lemba and Mosphilia.

Some individuals could not be assigned a definite age but it was possible to allocate them to the various age groups. These individuals were proportionately included into their appropriate age groups, explaining the appearance of fractions in Table 4.1. Infants from Souskiou and Lemba appear to be under-represented (see Figure 4.1 for comparison with model life table). With Souskiou, this may be due to either the destruction of infant remains from the many years of looting or the failure of the excavators to take notice of the smaller infant bones. While Lemba has no evidence of looting, the low infant numbers may be representative of sampling or a lower probability of burial of infants. The figures for the children are too small to draw definite conclusions. The presence of children and infants in the cemetery is evidence they (at least some of them) were considered full members of the society and therefore were permitted to be buried along with the adults.

	SOU		KM			
Age Class	Deaths	%	Deaths	%	Deaths	%
I (0-11 mo)	3	7.9	16	20.5	6	11.5
C1 (1-6)	3.5	9.2	26.5	34	23	44.2
C2 (7-12)	0.5	1.3	4.5	5.8	3	5.8
SA (13-18)	6	15.8	5.5	7.1	5	9.6
A1 (19-30)	16.7	43.9	10.8	13.9	7	13.5
A2 (31-45)	6	15.7	9.8	12.6	7	13.5
A3 (46+)	2.3	6.3	4.8	6.2	1	1.9
	38	**100**	**78**	**100**	**52**	**100**

Table 4.2 – Mortality of Southwest Cyprus

The second age group (1-6) has a similar pattern, Souskiou again has the lowest number, Lemba and Mosphilia with much higher numbers. The same reasons for Souskiou, mentioned above, may apply here as well, while Mosphilia may have a lower number due to sampling. The child group (7-12) is low in all three sites, which is expected according to life model tables (Coale and Demeny 1983).

4.2.5 ADULT MORTALITY

Lemba and Mosphilia have similar patterns all through the data of the age at death (Table 4.2) (Figure 4.1). The differences between these two sites and Souskiou may have much to do with sampling error and the looting, which occurred at the site. In Figure 4.1, the thick line represents the mortality profile calculated from the model life table West series (Coale and Demeny 1983) with a life expectancy at birth of thirty (E=30). The importance of the added life model data is explained well by Triantaphyllou:

> "The survivorship curves of the case study burial assemblages provide an additional visual aid to comparing several assemblages with the model life table. According to the E_{30} life model, survivorship should decline sharply in first two age categories, neonates and infants, followed by a slight decrease from childhood and prime adulthood, and then a renewed sharp decline in old age." (Triantaphyllou, 2001:37-41)

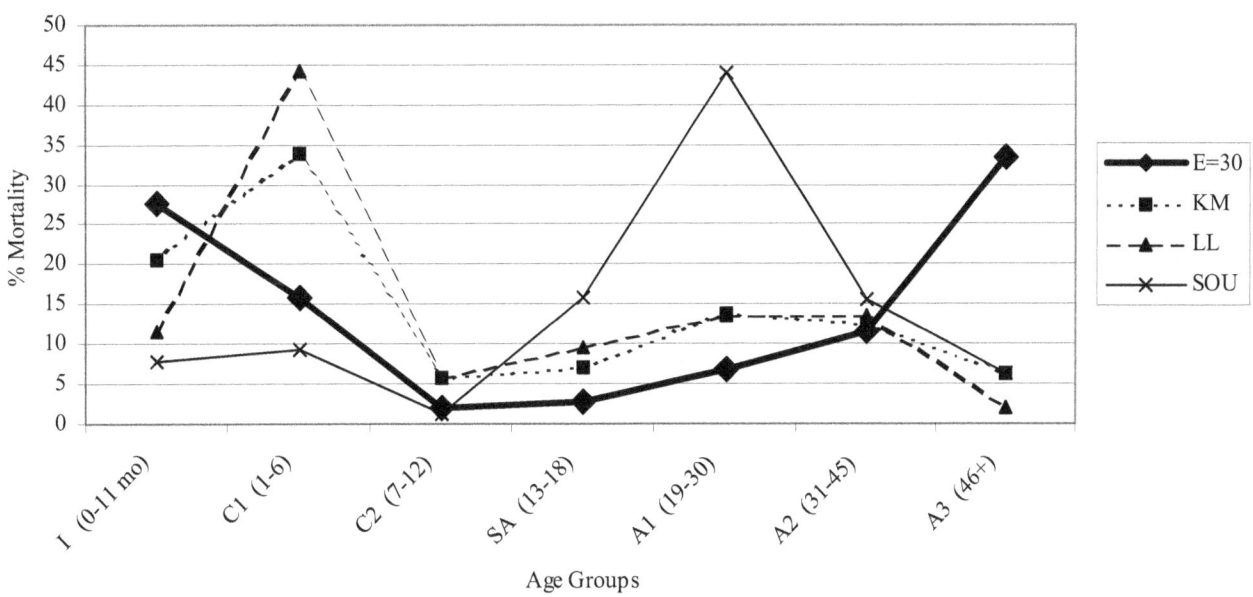

Figure 4.1 – Southwest Cyprus Mortality Profile and E=30

Since the samples in this study are from archaeological assemblages and not complete, comparing them to the West series data from Coale and Demeny (1983) can show where the archaeological data is missing individuals from each age group. Using the age at death of thirty has been a baseline human demographic pattern with which to compare the overall shape of the distribution because it is an average age at death for most prehistoric populations (Gage 2000; Triantaphyllou, 2001). From the many populations studied by Angel has determined the average age at death for ancient Mediterranean people is approximately thirty years (Angel 1945; 1946; 1969; 1970; 1977).

Mosphilia has the largest samples and the highest averages in all of the adult categories, except for the male age at death, which is slightly higher than Souskiou (Table 4.3). The average age at death for males from all three sites are similar, with Souskiou having the highest value of 35.5 years (No. 5). The main difference in age is between the female age at death ranging from 24 – 34. The low age from Souskiou is possibly due to sampling error.

Adults	SOU	No.	LL	No.	KM	No.
Avg. Age at Death	29.9	21	31.2	15	33.6	23
Avg. Age at Death Female	24.2	3	27	8	34.9	12
Avg. Age at Death Male	35.5	5	34.9	5	33.3	9
Avg. only F and M	31.2	8	30	13	34.2	21

Table 4.3 – Adult Mortality of Southwest Cyprus

The trend with the three sites is for more females dying in the first adult age group. This age group (as well as the 13-18 adolescent age group) is the child-bearing years when many women die during childbirth (Şenyürek 1947). This high mortality rate keeps the female average age low. Out of the 22 adults who died in the first age group (from all sites) 13 are female while only 9 are male. In the second age group, more females than males died.

The survivorship graph (Figure 4.2) again shows Souskiou may be under-represented in children and has a more dramatic peak in the first child group (1-6). Compared with E=30 even Lemba and Mosphilia show signs of being under-represented in children. Lemba and Mosphilia seem to match each other almost equally throughout the graph. This similarity may have more to do with both these sites having similar burial practices as the archaeologists did an excellent job in finding and excavating most of the human remains. Therefore both groups of human remains may represent adequate samples from the overall population.

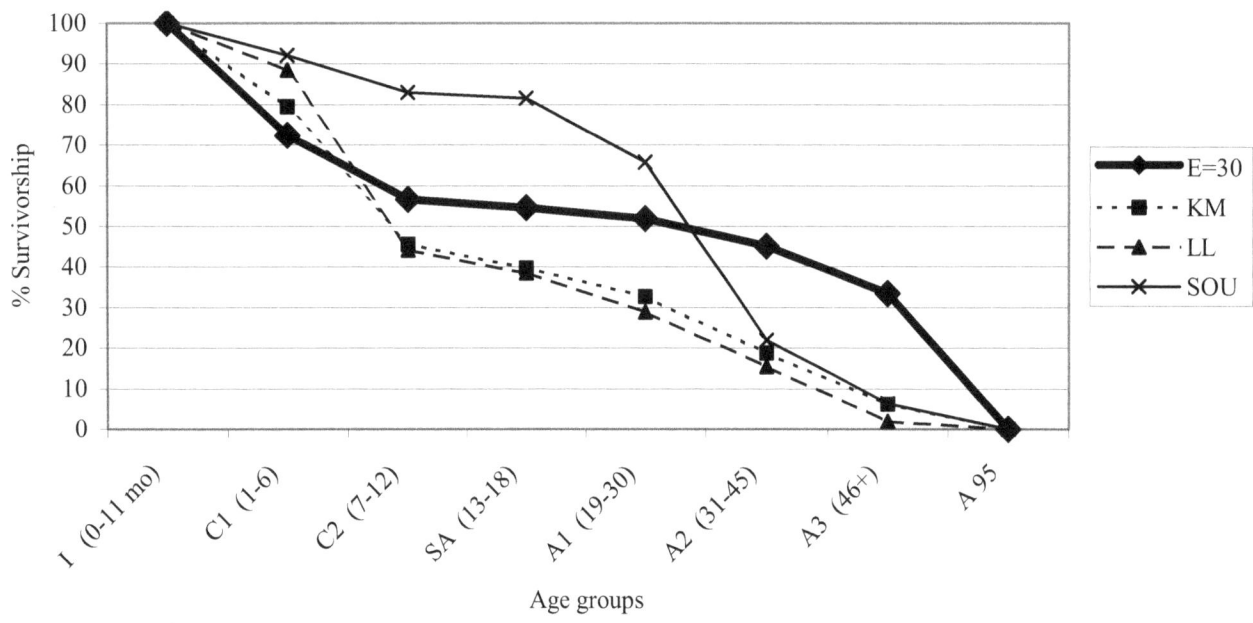

Figure 4.2 – Survivorship of Southwest Cyprus and E=30

4.2.6 KOLMOGOROV-SMIRNOV TEST

The Kolmogorov-Smirnov significance test was performed on the percentage of deaths in each age group between 2 samples. For this test it is recommended each sample should be greater than 40 in number, but Souskiou was still included even though there are only 38 individuals in the sample (Shennan 1997). The null hypothesis for this test is each of the two samples came from similar populations and the difference is only chance variation. This test presupposes the samples are chosen at random. Table 4.4 shows all of the results from the test on all of the paired comparisons in this chapter.

According to the Kolmogorov-Smirnov test, when Souskiou is compared with Lemba and Mosphilia, the greatest difference lies with the C2 (7-12) age group. By the end of the C2 age group 18% of individuals from Souskiou are dead compared to 62% and 60% of individuals from Lemba and Mosphilia, respectively (Table 4.4). This difference is significant at the 0.05 level suggesting these samples are from different populations. This suggests the sample from Souskiou under-represents children.

The test between Lemba and Mosphilia shows the greatest difference between the two samples lies in the I (0-11 mo) age group. By the end of this age group, 12% of individuals from Lemba and 21% of individuals from Mosphilia are dead. The sample from Lemba may under-represent children compared with Mosphilia. This difference is not significant at the 0.05 level suggesting these samples could be from the same population. Regarding the Mortality graph (Figure 4.1) and the Survivorship curve (Figure 4.2), Lemba and Mosphilia follow each other very closely, while Souskiou is clearly different.

Sample	Deaths (%)	Sample	Deaths (%)	Difference (%)	Age Group
SOU	18	LL	62	43	C2 (7-12)
SOU	18	KM	60	42	C2 (7-12)
SOU	8	Khirokitia	39	31	I (0-11mo)
LL	12	KM	21	9*	I (0-11mo)
LL	12	Khirokitia	39	27	I (0-11mo)
KM	21	Khirokitia	39	18*	I (0-11mo)
JT	59	Karataş	18	40	C1 (1-6)
LER	36	AS	54	19	I (0-11mo)
LER	59	Kephala	22	38	SA (13-18)
AS	76	Kephala	22	54	SA (13-18)
AI	0	EN	9	8*	C1 (1-6)

Table 4.4 – Kolmogorov-Smirnov Test for all comparisons. All Difference (%) numbers are significant at the 0.05 level (* Not significant at the 0.05 level)

4.2.7 OTHER CYPRIOT SITES

There are very few samples of human remains for this time period from Cyprus, therefore assemblages of human remains adjacent to the time periods of the three sites will be compared. The site of Sotira-Teppes is located approximately 20 km due east of Souskiou and north of the Limassol coast (Dikaios 1961; Niklasson 1991).

Sotira is a ceramic Neolithic (4500-3800 BC) site whose time period partly overlaps with Souskiou. Sotira has a small sample of human remains studied by J. Lawrence Angel, with only one child and 7 adults (five males and two females) (Angel 1961). The child has an age of 4 years and the five males have an average age at death of 38.6 years. The two females have an average age at death of 31 years. The breakdown for each age group is just as limiting as the average age at death for both sexes. The five males are all in the second age group (31-45) with the oldest male being 43 years of age. For the females, there is only one in the first and second age groups with the oldest female being 42 years of age. The combined average of these seven adults is 36.4 years. These numbers are very small and limiting for what can be learned, when compared to Souskiou, Lemba and Mosphilia. The female average for Sotira is higher than Lemba or Souskiou, and lower than Mosphilia, but the small sample size of two individuals does not make this comparison significant. On the other hand, the male average from Sotira is very high compared with these three sites. Comparing such a small sample as Sotira to these three sites does not lead to any conclusions of demographic patterns, but has been mentioned for completeness.

The site of Khirokitia-Vounoi is located approximately 65 km due east of Souskiou, also relatively near the coast (Map 2) (Dikaios 1953). This is an aceramic Neolithic site, which is much older than Souskiou. The time range for this site is >6000-5200 BC (Niklasson 1991). It is remarkable for the great number of human remains from such an ancient site. The remains were studied by J. Lawrence Angel (1953; 1961), R.-P. Charles (1962), G. Kurth (1958; 1980) and from a recent excavation, by F. Le Mort (2000). The data compared in this study comes from the data compiled by K. Niklasson up to the publication of that work (Niklasson 1991). An additional 27 burials were uncovered from further excavations during the 1970's, which were not available for inclusion in the 1991 publication. There was enough data to create a mortality table from the data extrapolated by the author from the available publications (Angel 1953; 1961; Niklasson 1991).

The Infant age group (0-11 mo) from Khirokitia has a very high infant mortality rate, much higher than those from the three much younger southwest Cypriot sites (Table 4.5). Comparing all of the childhood years from birth until 12 years of age (the first 3 age groups), the combined percentages are more informative. The combined percentage of Khirokitia is 45.8%, Mosphilia is 60.3%, Lemba is slightly higher with 61.5% and Souskiou is much lower at 18.4%. In actuality the mortality rate for children from Khirokitia is much lower than sites from a much younger period in Cyprus' history. While Khirokitia may be well represented in the first age group, it seems to be under-represented in the other 2 child age groups, possibly due to sampling error.

Age Class	Deaths	%
I (0-11 mo)	64	38.6
C1 (1-6)	10	6
C2 (7-12)	2	1.2
SA (13-18)	8	4.8
A1 (19-30)	38.2	23
A2 (31-45)	34.3	20.7
A3 (46+)	9.5	5.7
	166	100

Table 4.5 – Mortality of Khirokitia-Vounoi (Modified from Niklasson 1991)

The combined adult average age of 34.4 years (No. 36) (Table 4.6) is higher than the age from Souskiou, Lemba and Mosphilia (Table 4.3). The average age for females is 32.3 years (No. 17), which is higher than Souskiou and Lemba but just under the average for Mosphilia. The male average age is the highest at 36.3 years (No. 19). With such a large sample from Khirokitia, the adult averages are significant.

Adults	Average	No.
Avg. Age at Death Female	32.29	17
Avg. Age at Death Male	36.26	19
Avg. Age at Death	34.39	36

Table 4.6 – Khirokitia-Vounoi Adult Mortality (Modified from Niklasson 1991)

The mortality graph presents what was already mentioned about the higher infant mortality from Khirokitia, the Child 1 (1-6) age group shows Khirokitia is under-represented in children (Figure 4.3). Souskiou has a higher percentage than Khirokitia. Khirokitia appears to follow the E=30 line on the survivorship graph except for the Adult 2 and Adult 3 age groups (Figure 4.4).

4.2.8 KOLMOGOROV-SMIRNOV TEST

According to the Kolmogorov-Smirnov test for Souskiou and Khirokitia, the difference between the two samples lies between the I (0-11 mo) age group and is 0.31 or 31% (Table 4.4). By the end of this age group 8% of individuals from Souskiou are dead and 39% of individuals from Khirokitia are dead. This suggests the sample from Souskiou is under-represented in children. This difference is significant at the 0.05 level suggesting these samples are from different populations.

The Kolmogorov-Smirnov test for Lemba and Khirokitia shows the difference between the two samples lies between the I (0-11 mo) age group and is 0.27 or 27%. By the end of this age group 12% of individuals from Lemba are dead and 39% of individuals from Khirokitia are dead. This difference is significant at the 0.05 level suggesting these samples are from different populations.

According to the Kolmogorov-Smirnov test for Mosphilia and Khirokitia, the difference between the two samples lies between the I (0-11 mo) age group and is 0.18 or 18%. By the end of the I age group 21% of individuals from Souskiou are dead and 39% of individuals from Khirokitia are dead. This suggests the sample from Souskiou under-represents children. This difference is not significant at the 0.05 level suggesting these samples could be from the same population. This may also mean the evidence is insufficient to suggest they are different.

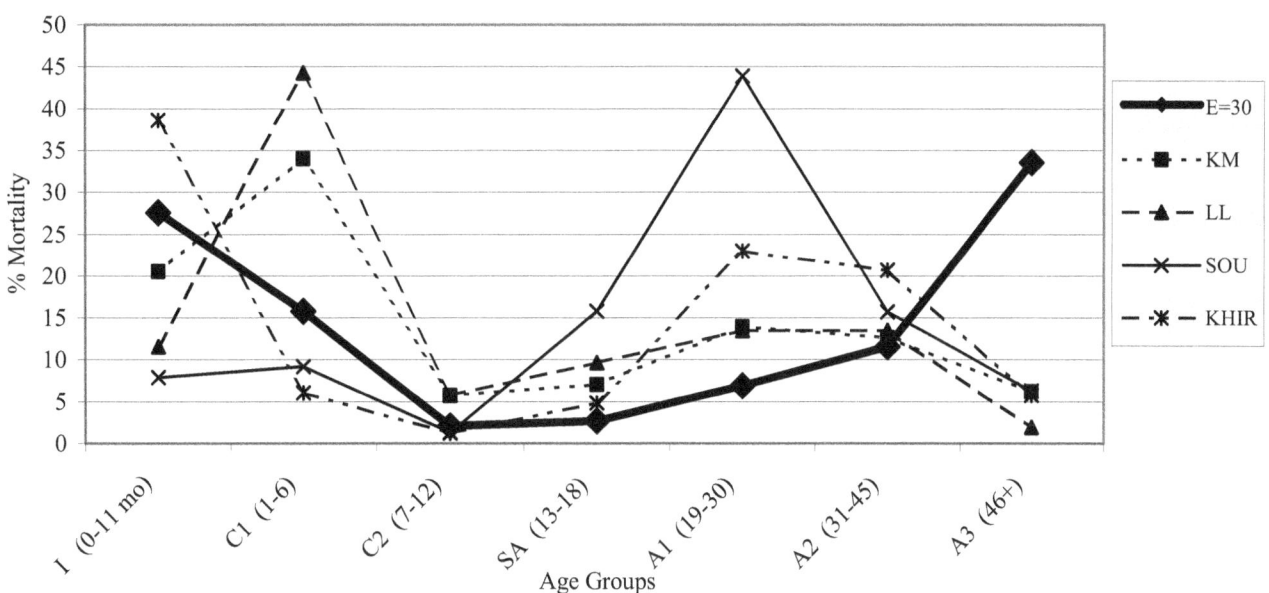

Figure 4.3 – Mortality profiles for southwest Cyprus and Khirokitia

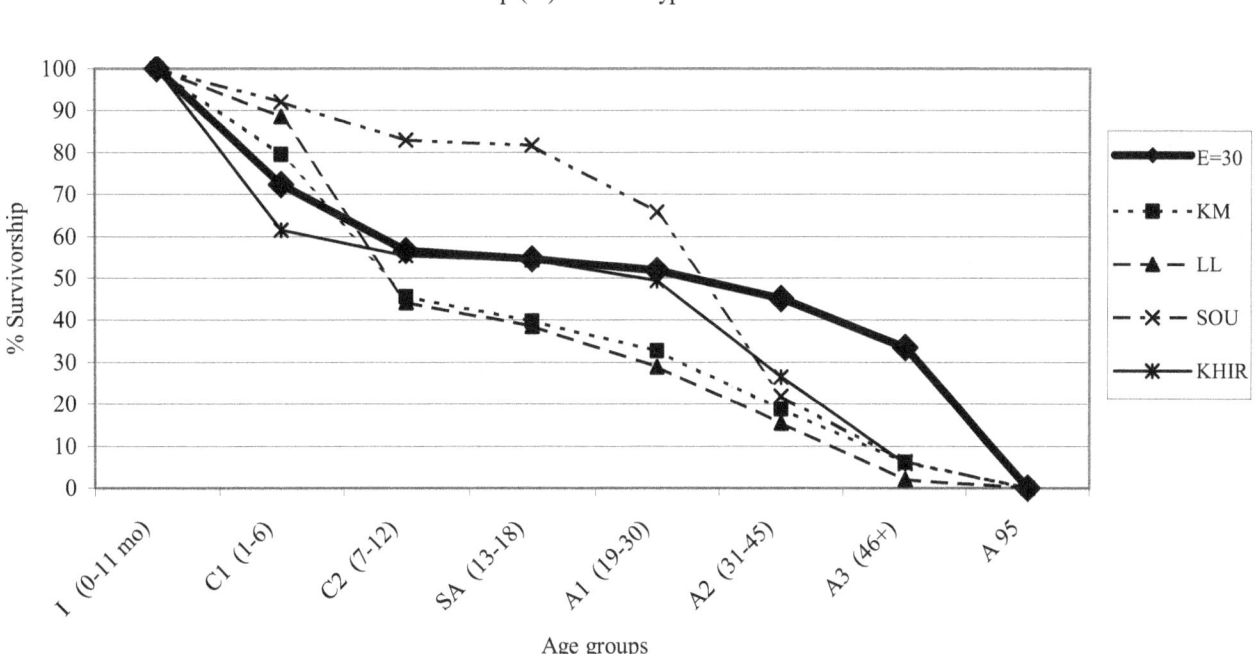

Figure 4.4 – Survivorship of southwest Cyprus and Khirokitia.

4.2.9 SUMMARY

There are some similarities in demography between Lemba and Mosphilia. Souskiou is deficient in numbers of infants, children and older adults. The comparison of the Neolithic site of Khirokitia to southwest Cyprus is not very informative since it also lacks infants.

4.3 REGIONAL COMPARISON
4.3.1 JERABLUS-TAHTANI

The next comparison will be with two other sites in the region, Jerablus in Syria and Karataş-Semayük in Turkey.

The skeletal remains studied are from a total of 44 tombs and from the excavation period 1992-1998. Dorothy A. Lunt and Marie E. Watt of the Department of Oral Sciences, University of Glasgow already published the preliminary report on these human remains (Peltenburg et al. 1995). Due to the fragmentary condition of the skeletal remains Drs. Lunt and Watt studied only the dentition. For this study there was enough skeletal material present for an anthropological study.

From the tombs studied, a MNI of 123 has been identified. The majority of the individuals come from the tombs surrounding Tomb 302 where 31 individuals have been identified. Due to the heavily disturbed nature of Tomb 302 the MNI is an estimate. The condition of the skeletal remains varied relative to the types of tombs they were in. The chamber tombs, such as Tomb 302 yielded very fragmentary remains but the smaller tombs and the pithos burials had many more complete bones. Foetuses were also discovered in some of the smaller burials.

4.3.2 JERABLUS-TAHTANI MORTALITY

Some individuals could not be assigned a definite age but it was possible to allocate them to the various age groups. These individuals were proportionately included into their appropriate age groups, explaining the appearance of fractions in Table 4.7. The site's demographic breakdown is typical of what one would expect with any prehistoric society, namely high rates of infant mortality with more people living into their twenties and fewer people living to old age (Gage 2000) (Figure 4.5).

Included in the Infant age group (from birth to 11 months after birth), are five foetuses aged from 7.5 to 9.5 months. These ages are on a 10 lunar month scale where birth can occur between 9 and 10 months (Kósa 1989). These foetuses were most likely premature births or stillborn. The foetuses are from tombs 1362, 1367, 1369, 1481 and Unit 1416. The combined number of infants and children represent approximately 63% of the entire sample. This is the expected proportion for a prehistoric community (Gage 2000).

4.3.3 ANATOLIA

The EBA site of Karataş-Semayük (2700 – 2300 B.C.), in the southwest region of Turkey, has a substantial number of human burials (Angel 1968; 1970). This site is a considerable distance from the Euphrates River Valley, but its usefulness is due to the similar time period as well as a large sample of human burials.

Out of a total of 540 individuals the combined infants and children make up only 33% of the entire sample (Table 4.7). According to Angel the low infant numbers suggest these people buried their infants outside of the regular cemetery (Angel 1968; 1970). Regarding the smaller population from Jerablus, the higher infant and child percentage, from the Syrian site, is better represented for a prehistoric population.

	JT		KS	
Age Class	Deaths	%	Deaths	%
I (0-11 mo)	49	39.8	31	5.8
C1 (1-6)*	23	18.7	66	12.4
C2 (7-12)	6	4.9	79	14.8
SA (13-18)	4	3.3	30	5.6
A1 (19-30)	21	17.1	136.4	25.5
A2 (31-45)	12.9	10.5	164.5	30.8
A3 (46+)	7.1	5.8	27.1	5.1
	123	100	534	100

Table 4.7 – Mortality of Jerablus (JT) and Karataş-Semayük (KS) (modified from Angel 1970) *Angel's children age is group is 1-4 years of age.

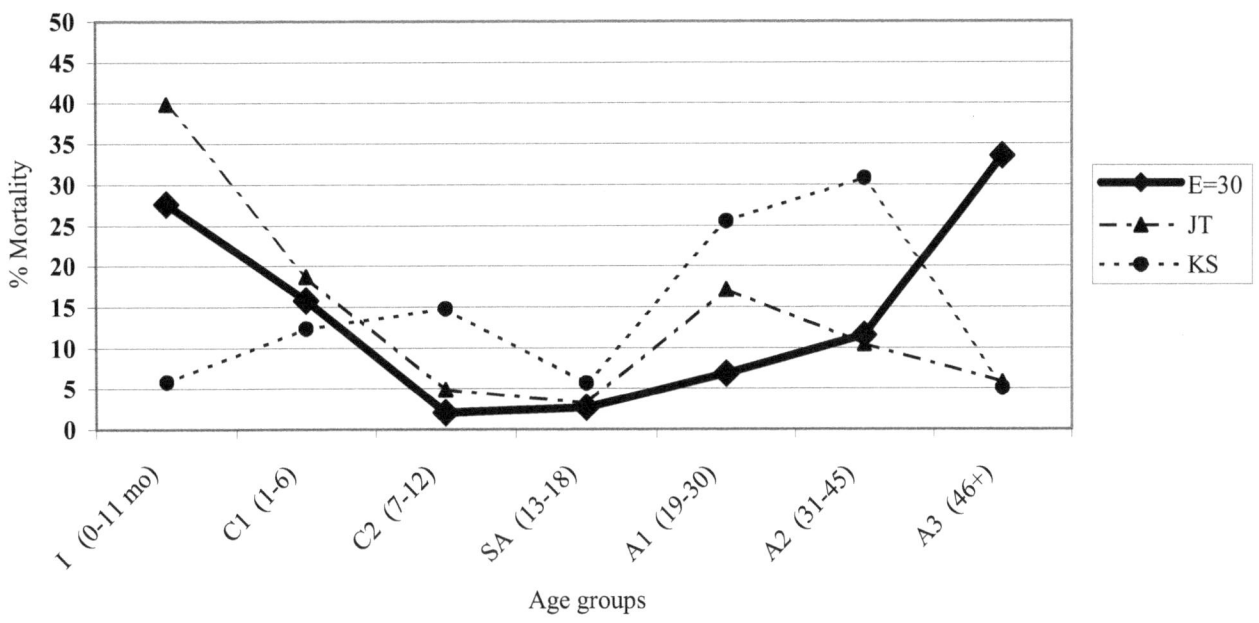

Figure 4.5 – Mortality of Jerablus, Karataş-Semayük and E=30

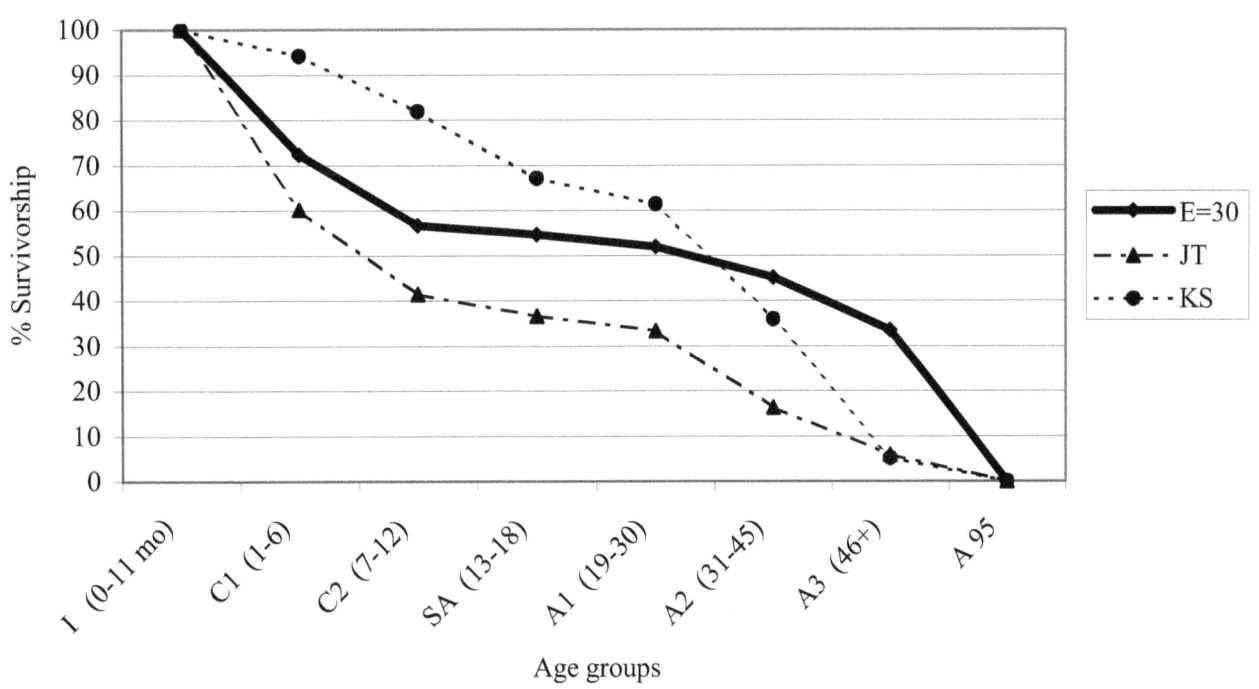

Figure 4.6 – Survivorship for Jerablus, Karataş-Semayük and E=30

The distribution of deaths between Jerablus and Karataş-Semayük is evident from the mortality graph (Figure 4.5). Jerablus closely follows E=30 except where it has more deaths in the first adult age group and too few in the last age group. While Karataş-Semayük clearly does not follow either data points, only the sub-adult data is similar. The survivorship data also supports the evidence in which the Karataş-Semayük sample is under-represented in people younger than the first adult age group (Figure 4.6).

4.3.4 ADULT MORTALITY FOR SYRIA AND ANATOLIA

From Jerablus in the first adult age group (19-30) there are nine male deaths and only four females. In the second age group, there are 3 males and 8 females. In the third age group there are 2 males and 2 females. Most populations in this study have shown more females die in the first adult age group. However in the case of Jerablus there are more males, keeping the male average age at death much lower than of the female average (Table 4.8). The male average is still higher than other sites in this study where the females have a lower average age. This suggests the females were living longer and the males were not living longer than males from other sites.

At Karataş-Semayük in Turkey, the average age at death for males is 33.8 (No. 143), while the female average is 29.8 (No. 190) (Angel 1970). From the adults aged 20 and over, 54.8% are females. Females also make up the largest number of deaths from 20-34 years of age (this group makes up 70.5% of all females, as opposed to 54.7% of males in the same age group) (Angel 1970). Males in the age range of 35-59 make up the higher percentage of the adult population (45.3% of all males are in this group as opposed to 29.5 % of all females). Karataş-Semayük is a larger sample than Jerablus and is probably more accurate for a prehistoric population, but it is clear the trend for adults from Jerablus is the opposite of Karataş-Semayük.

Adults	JT	No.	KS	No.
Avg. Age at Death	33.5	40	31.8	324
Avg. Age at Death Female	36.3	13	29.8	190
Avg. Age at Death Male	31	14	33.8	134
Avg. only F & M	33.5	27	31.8	324

Table 4.8 - Jerablus and Karataş-Semayük Adult Mortality (From Angel 1968)

The Turkish anthropologist Muzaffer Süleyman Şenyürek has studied many human remains from sites throughout Turkey. Şenyürek has noted throughout the Turkish Chalcolithic and Early Bronze Age is the low infant mortality numbers, which he suggests should be higher due to the difficulty in finding and recovering infant and children's remains (Şenyürek 1947). This evidence is reflected in the infant and child mortality percentages from Lemba and Mosphilia, which are over 50% (Table 4.2).

Şenyürek also notes even with small samples the percentage of old age deaths does not differ from the 4th millennium B.C. up to the middle 1st millennium B.C. Only with the Roman-Byzantine sample (1st millennium A.D.) does the percentage increase significantly (Şenyürek 1947). This suggests a long established demographic pattern within Anatolia. This continuity has also been noticed on Cyprus from the Neolithic to the Chalcolithic.

Şenyürek (1947) also mentions ancient Anatolian females do have higher mortality in the early periods of life (Şenyürek also includes the sub-adult category 13-20 years). He suggests this difference in mortality rates is directly related to the childbearing period, the difference due to the hazards of child bearing (Şenyürek 1947). This trend has also been identified on Cyprus and in other sites around Anatolia already mentioned in this study. Only Jerablus seems to have a different pattern with regard to the adult age at death.

4.3.5 KOLMOGOROV-SMIRNOV TEST

The Kolmogorov-Smirnov test between Jerablus and Karataş-Semayük shows the difference between the two samples lies with the first child age group (1-6) at 0.40 or 40% (Table 4.4). By the end of this age group 40% of individuals from Jerablus are dead and 18% of individuals from Karataş-Semayük are dead. These results suggest the sample from Karataş-Semayük is under-represented in children. This difference is significant at the 0.05 level suggesting these samples are from different populations.

4.3.6 SUMMARY

The high infant mortality common for most prehistoric populations is not evident from Karataş-Semayük, while Jerablus does exhibit the usual pattern also observed on Cyprus. The pattern observed thus far with regards to the average age at death for females has been lower than males, although at Jerablus this is the opposite. This difference may be due to sampling error, or it may have more to do with the health of the people from the site.

4.4 AEGEAN SITES

This section includes data from two sites from which were collected from the Greek mainland sites of Lerna and Asine. The Greek sites of Ayios Kosmas and Kephala will also be included as a comparison.

4.4.1 ASINE

The remains from Asine were collected from 77 tombs. Fürst (1930) and Angel (1982) previously studied the human remains. An anthropological study is currently being conducted by Anne Ingvarsson-Sundström from Uppsala University, Sweden as part of her PhD thesis. She was kind enough to share the anthropological data she compiled on the remains. I travelled to the University of Uppsala to study the collection of human remains and included the age and sex data Anne Ingvarsson-Sundström had already compiled.

4.4.2 LERNA

The skeletal remains were from a total of 228 tombs and studied by J. Lawrence Angel (1971). Angel completed a very thorough anthropological study on the remains, which were compared to the data collected. The excellent and systematic excavation conducted by Jack Caskey and the American School of Classical Studies in the 1950's uncovered a great deal of skeletal remains (Caskey 1954, 1955, 1956, 1957, 1958, 1959, 1960). The MNI for this sample is 229 individuals, the largest number of all the sites in this study; hence it is a very good size for analysis and comparison.

4.4.3 AYIOS KOSMAS

Ayios Kosmas is an EBA settlement and cemetery in Attica, with the cemeteries belonging to the EH period (Mylonas 1934; 1959). The site was excavated from the end of the 19th century until the 1950's (Mylonas 1959). The human remains in this study are from the excavations carried out in the 1930's and the 1950's and were studied by J. Lawrence Angel (Angel 1959).

The 35 remains from Ayios Kosmas have indicated small body size and both wiry and stocky build with considerable population variety (Angel 1959; 1971). Out of the 35 people excavated from the site only the 25 adults will be included in this study, as there are not enough children for a proper demographic comparison.

4.4.4 KEPHALA

The site of Kephala on the island of Keos in the Aegean is a Late Neolithic site and is included in this study because of its adequate sample size for comparison (Angel 1977). The site was excavated by a team lead by John Coleman in the 1960's and 1970's and J. Lawrence Angel studied the human remains (Angel 1977). The settlement is dated to the late 4th millennium B.C. (3300-3200 B.C.) and lasted roughly one to two centuries (Coleman 1977).

4.4.5 GREEK MORTALITY

The largest numbers of individuals from prehistoric sites are usually children, due to high infant mortality. Nowhere is this more evident than at Asine, which has a very high infant mortality rate (Table 4.9). At Lerna the infant group is lower and out of these 82 deaths in the first age group, 39 of the infants died within the first month of life. According to Angel the low infant number from Kephala suggests most newborn infants who died prematurely were not buried formally and were excluded from the cemetery. This would explain the low infant numbers (Table 4.9) (Angel 1977).

	AS		LER		KE	
Age Class	Deaths	%	Deaths	%	Deaths	%
I (0-11mo)	79	54.5	82	35.8	5	7.7
C1 (>1-6)	21	14.5	39	17.0	5.7	8.8
C2 (7-12)	6	4.1	7	3.1	2.3	3.5
SA (13-18)	4	2.8	8	3.5	1	1.5
A1 (19-30)	21	14.5	34.1	14.9	27.9	43
A2 (31-45)	14	9.7	50.6	22.1	23.1	35.5
A3 (46+)	0	0	8.3	3.6	0	0
	145	100	229	100	65	100

Table 4.9 – Mortality of Asine, Lerna and Kephala (Angel 1977)

Relative to the number of infants, the number of children from Asine is still high but significantly lower. At Lerna the number is slightly higher although lower than Kephala. The numbers for all three sites begin to decline in the second child age group (7-12) and well into the sub-adult age group (13-18) (Figure 4.7). The number of individuals who died in the sub-adults age group seems to stabilise, which is what one would expect with a prehistoric population.

The number of deaths for all three sites starts to increase with the first adult age group (19-30). An interesting note about the adult data is there are no survivors into the oldest age group from Asine and Kephala. The oldest ages the adults reached from Asine were 40, 40 and 45 years. It is interesting to note even in a wealthy and prosperous community such as Lerna, the number of people living beyond 45 years of age is quite small.

The distribution of deaths in Greek samples is evident when looking at the mortality and survivorship graphs (Figure 4.7 & Figure 4.8). Kephala is under-represented in children while Asine is under-represented in adults. The sample from Lerna is better represented in all age groups and follows E=30 closely until the last two adult age groups where it also drops away, having too few adults.

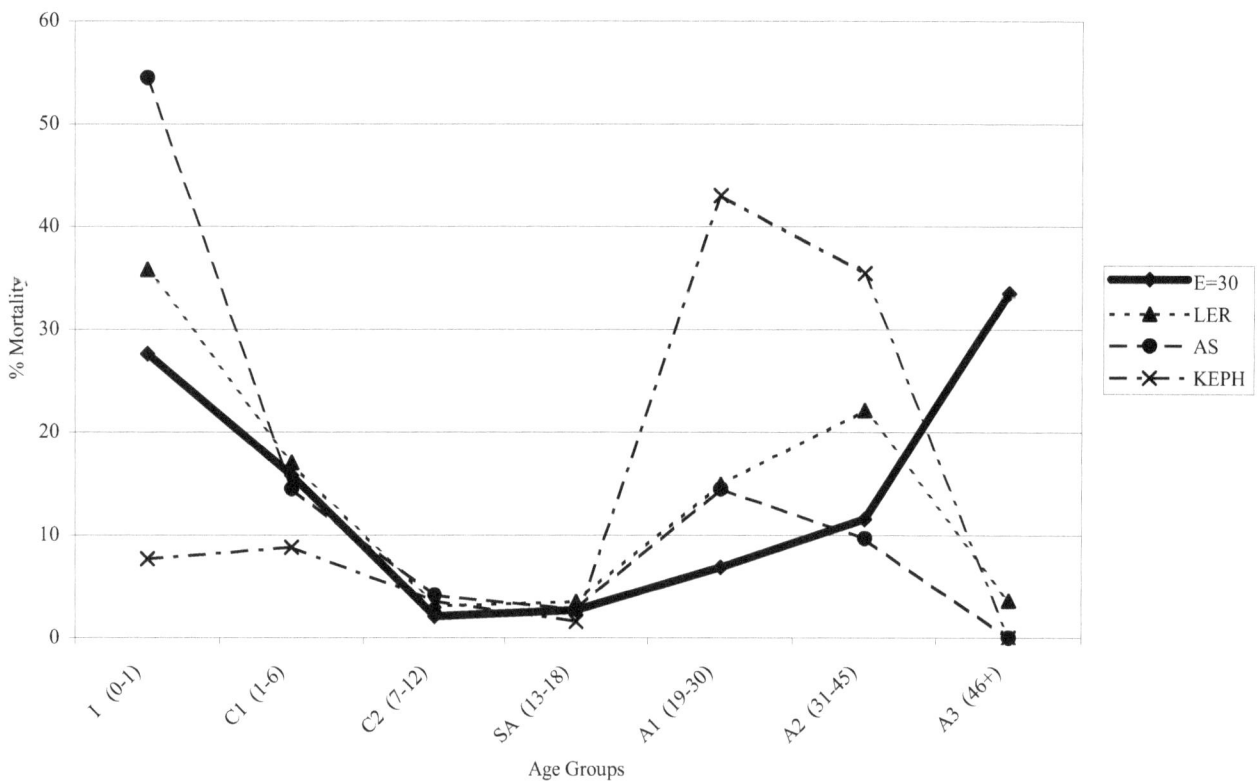

Figure 4.7 – Mortality of Lerna, Asine, Kephala and E=30

4.4.6 ADULT MORTALITY FOR GREECE

Although there are 145 individuals from Asine, most are children with only ten adults of known age from which to determine sex. The average age at death for all ten adults from Asine is 31 years of age. The age for the only female is 20 years and the two males come to an average of 40 years of age (Table 4.10). With such small numbers there can be no significant conclusion drawn from them, except perhaps males had a longer life span than females. According to Angel, the male average age at death was 35 years and the female average was 30 years (Angel 1982).

This trend continues for the remaining three sites, with males living longer than females (Table 4.10). Lerna has the oldest male age while Kephala and Ayios Kosmas are almost identical. The range between males and females for the three sites is between 5.3 to 6.3 years. The same pattern of more females dying in the first adult age group is also evident with these three sample (Table 4.11).

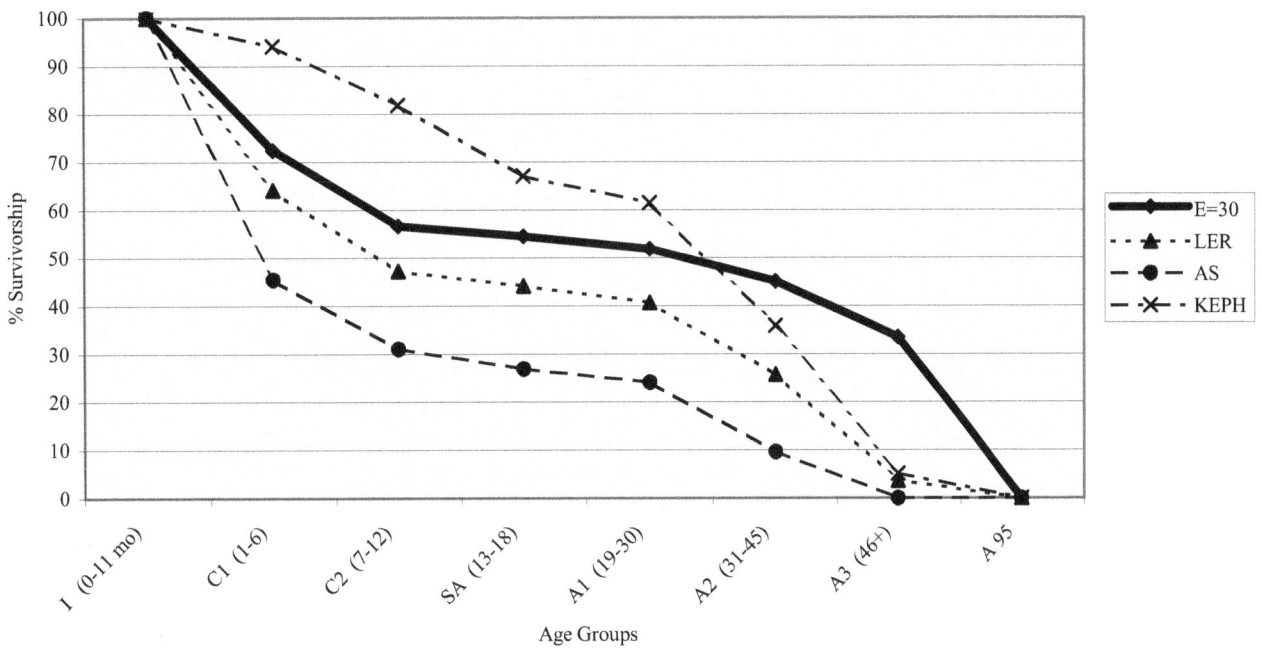

Figure 4.8 – Survivorship for Asine, Lerna, Kephala and E=30

Adults	AS	No.	LER	No.	KE	No.	AK	No.
Avg Age at Death	31	10	34.7	92	31	39	32.7	25
Avg Age at Death Female	20	1	31.7	40	28	21	29	9
Avg Age at Death Male	40	2	37.1	51	34.5	18	34.8	16
Avg only F and M	33	3	34.7	91	31.1	39	32.7	25

Table 4.10 – Adult Mortality of Asine, Lerna, Kephala (KE) and Ayios Kosmas (AK).

	LER		AK		KE	
	M	F	M	F	M	F
A1(19-30)	12	21	6	7	5	16
A2(31-45)	32	16	9	2	13	5
A3(46+)	7	1	1	0	0	0

Table 4.11 – Breakdown by sex of adults from Greece (LER=Lerna, AK=Ayios Kosmas, KE=Kephala).

4.4.7 KOLMOGOROV-SMIRNOV TEST

According to the Kolmogorov-Smirnov test for Asine and Lerna, the difference between the two samples lies with the I (0-11 mo) age group and is 0.19. By the end of the I age group 54% of individuals from Asine are dead and 36% of individuals from Lerna are dead (Table 4.4). This could suggest Lerna is under-represented in infants, compared with Asine.

The difference with Kephala and Lerna is in the sub-adult age group (13-18) and is 0.38. By the end of this age group,

22% of individuals from Kephala are dead and 59% of individuals from Lerna are dead. The results from Asine are similar where the greatest difference with the two sites is also in the sub-adult age group (13-18) and is 0.54. By the end of this age group only 22% of individuals from Kephala are dead while from Asine 76% individuals are dead. This test adds to the evidence the sample from Kephala is under-represented in children relative to Asine and Lerna. The test results for these three sites are all significant at the 0.05 level suggesting these samples are from different populations.

4.4.8 SUMMARY

The sites described above have a similar demographic profile as the other sites examined in this study: high infant mortality, low age at death for adult females and a higher number of females dying in the first adult age group. The problem of under-represented infants and children is common from archaeological assemblages, as observed in the above samples.

4.5 LATE BRONZE AGE NORTHEAST CYPRUS

The following sites could have been included in the regional comparison with southwest Cyprus but as these sites are from the Late Bronze Age, I believe they were best suited to be used as temporal comparisons. As with southwest Cyprus during the Early Bronze Age, there are few samples of human remains to conduct a thorough comparison. The Late Bronze Age site of Hala Sultan Tekke, for example, has too few human remains to make a significant contribution to this analysis (Schwartz 1976). Therefore only the sites of Ayios Iakovos and Enkomi will be included in this comparison.

4.5.1 AYIOS IAKOVOS

This site is one of the two Late Bronze Age sites, which make up the northern Cypriot sample. Fürst (1933) and Fischer (1986) previously studied the human remains. The archaeological report from Gjerstad (et al. 1934) mentions there were communal tombs, containing only adults. Therefore, this sample is under-represented in sub-adults and children (Table 4.12). Fifteen individuals, who could not be located during the data collection, have been included in the demography table from the analysis done by Fürst (1933). This additional information came from two tombs, yielding fourteen individuals.

4.5.2 ENKOMI

The human remains are from nineteen tombs excavated during the Swedish Cypriot Expedition from 1927-1931 (Gjerstad 1934). Fürst (1933) and Hjortsjö (1946-7) previously studied the human remains. As with the previous site of Ayios Iakovos, eleven individuals, who could not be located for this study, have been included in the demography table from the analysis done by Fürst (1933).

4.5.3 MORTALITY

Both Enkomi and Ayios Iakovos are under-represented in children, affecting the overall percentage breakdown of the samples (Figure 4.9). The percentages of both of these sites come close to the E=30 population, suggesting that although under-represented, the normal pattern for these populations may be beginning with the sub-adults.

	AI		EN	
Age Class	Deaths	%	Deaths	%
I (0-11 mo)	0	0	0	0
C1 (1-6)	0	0	7	8.8
C2 (7-12)	3	6.7	3	3.8
SA (13-18)	3	6.7	1	1.3
A1 (19-30)	9.6	21.4	15.5	19.4
A2 (31-45)	22.6	50.2	37.8	47.2
A3 (46+)	6.8	15.1	15.7	19.6
	45	100	80	100

Table 4.12 – Mortality of Ayios Iakovos and Enkomi

The survivorship graph of the two sites also shows a dramatic difference from the E=30 data (Figure 4.10). These sites do follow each other quite closely and may be evidence of the type of cultural distinction occurring with the burial of these individuals. Clearly only a certain age group of the society is being buried in these large communal chamber tombs.

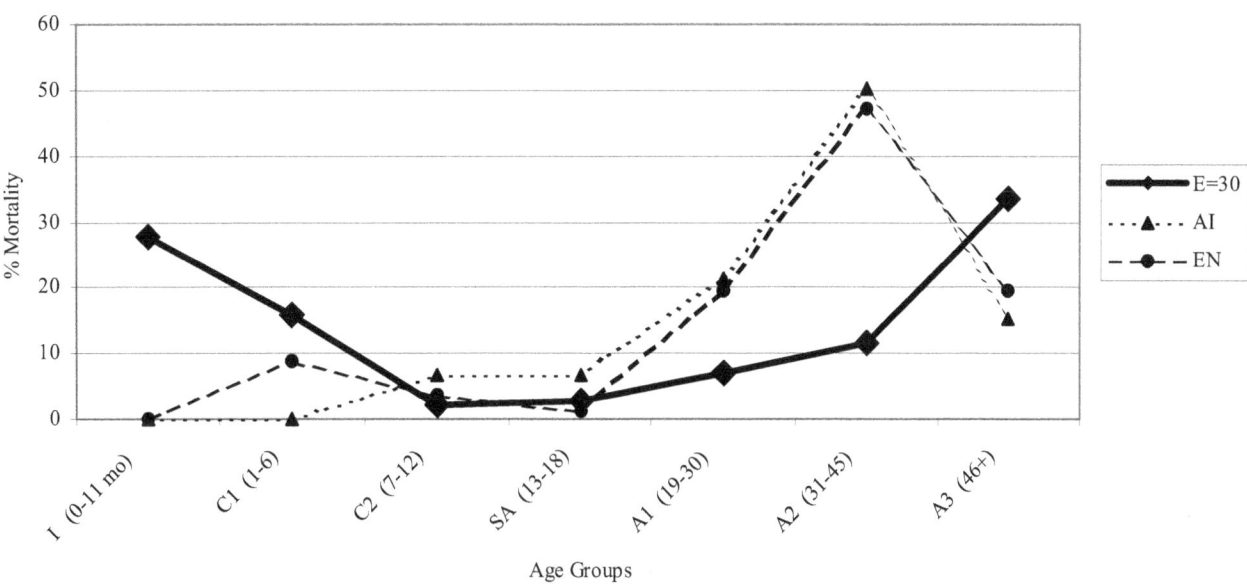

Figure 4.9 – Mortality of Enkomi, Ayios Iakovos and E=30

4.5.4 ADULT MORTALITY

The overall average age at death for adults is higher from Enkomi than from Ayios Iakovos (Table 4.13). The values from both sites are higher than the values observed from the more ancient sites in this chapter. Since both these sites have a large enough sample of adults, these ages should be considered significant.

Adults	AI	No.	EN	No.
Avg Age at Death	35.1	26	40.1	56
Avg Age at Death Female	33.2	10	36.1	23
Avg Age at Death Male	36.3	16	42.9	33

Table 4.13 – Adult Mortality of Ayios Iakovos and Enkomi

These two sites continue to show the same pattern observed from other samples in this chapter, with more females dying in the first adult age group (A1 19-30) than males. This pattern continues in the second adult age group (A2 31-45) with more male than female deaths. The final adult age group (A3 46+) shows a mixed pattern with more males than females from Enkomi while the number of deaths from Ayios Iakovos are equal (Table 4.14).

From Ayios Iakovos the oldest female is approximately 50 years and the oldest male is approximately 46 years. The opposite is true from Enkomi with the oldest male approximately 50 years and the oldest female is approximately 46 years of age.

	AI		EN	
	M	F	M	F
A1(19-30)	4	5	4	7
A2(31-45)	10	3	23	13
A3(46+)	2	2	6	2

Table 4.14 – Breakdown by sex of adults from Ayios Iakovos and Enkomi

4.5.5 KOLMOGOROV-SMIRNOV TEST

According to the Kolmogorov-Smirnov test results for Ayios Iakovos and Enkomi, the difference between the samples lies in the first child age group (1-6) and is 0.08 (Table 4.4). By the end of this age group 0% of the individuals from Ayios Iakovos are dead and 9% of individuals from Enkomi are dead. This difference is not significant at the 0.05 level suggesting these samples could be from the same population. It may also suggest there is insufficient evidence that they are different. It is more likely that the latter is true.

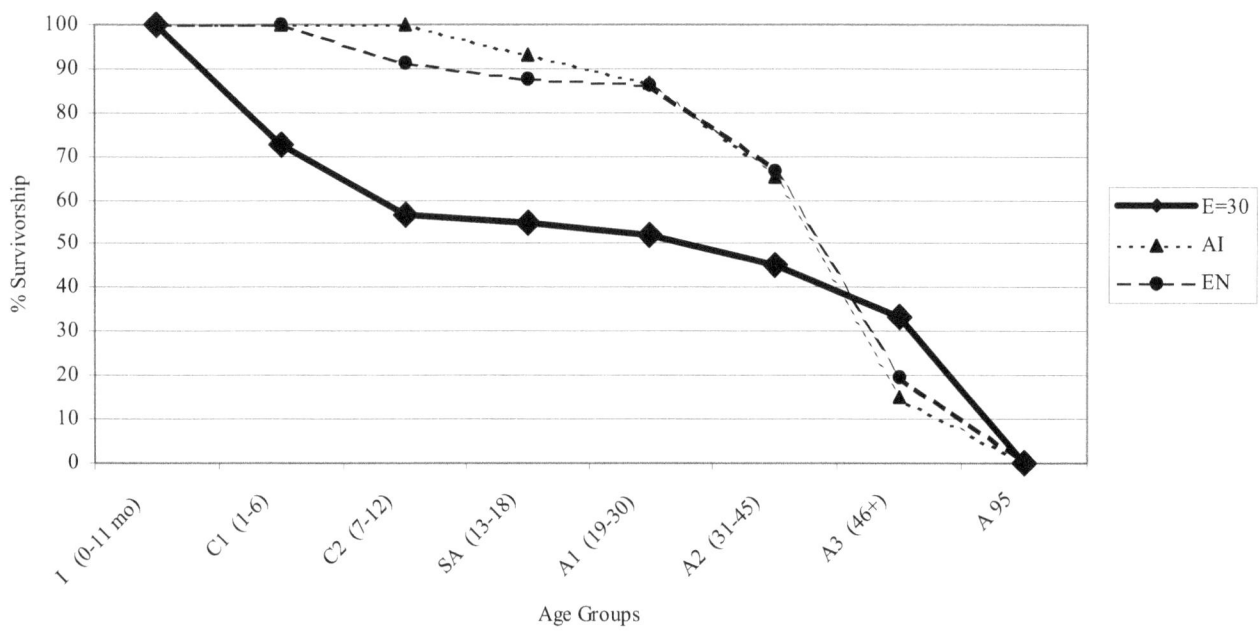

Figure 4.10 – Survivorship of northeast Cyprus and E=30

4.5.6 SUMMARY

These sites are under-represented in children and infants, which are probably due to the nature of the burials, rather than preservation or recovery techniques. Therefore, there is little which can be learned from that aspect of the demography. The adult data shows the same pattern observed in most the other sites, suggesting even from these assemblages, which are incomplete, they follow the expected pattern as with older sites. Also interesting to note is the increase in adult age at death compared to the older populations.

4.6 CHAPTER SUMMARY

Comparing the sites in this study, which have different excavation histories and are from different time periods poses a problem when comparing them. There is also the added complication of these sites having been excavated by different archaeologists and techniques throughout the 20th century. As with any archaeological assemblage these samples are incomplete which always affect the analysis.

4.6.1 SOUTHWEST CYPRUS

The demography from Lemba and Mosphilia are very similar, due to the type of sites and where the burials are located. Excavation of both by the University of Edinburgh adds to the consistency of the excavation methods and results. This suggests the demographic analysis from these two sites reflect the real demographic pattern of sites of that time and location. Souskiou, however, has a much more complicated excavation history that affects the demographic analysis. The post-mortem damage and extensive looting has affected the skeletal remains and recovery of bones. The post-mortem damage has also affected the condition of the teeth that represent the most durable aspect of the skeleton. The fact there are so few children located at the site could make this demographic analysis suspect. The lack of children also skews the percentage of adults from Souskiou, which may or may not be accurate. It is important to remember that Souskiou is a unique site in the history of Cyprus. The special location of this cemetery and social customs may be affecting the demographic distribution. Even with such small demographic samples it appears there is a difference in the demographic breakdown between these two types of sites that is likely due to social customs dictating the distribution of children and adults. Clearly, more cemetery sites with large samples are needed for more accurate analyses.

4.6.2 NORTHEAST CYPRUS

The samples from Ayios Iakovos and Enkomi share similarities in the excavation methods as the Swedish Expedition to Cyprus excavated both. As these two sites were not looted and did not suffer from the same post-mortem damage as Souskiou suggests they are representative of the actual demographic pattern. The only other factor that could affect the analysis is the standard anthropological practices used in the 1920's and 1930's when mostly long bones and skulls were collected and the remainder of the skeleton was not. In the case of children and infant bones, these were also ignored and possibly not identified due to the anthropological training during that era. It is clear that the archaeological methods clearly affect the demographic analysis of these two sites. Not knowing how much was not recovered from the chamber tombs will affect the validity of the data set.

4.6.3 GREECE

There are differences between the samples from Lerna and Asine that may affect the demographic analysis. As mentioned above, there are the differences between anthropological practices from the 1920's and the 1970's. It is clear there are some gaps in the sample that may be affecting the analysis. There is a marked lack of teeth for such a large number of individuals from the site, although the demographic breakdown appears to be consistent with prehistoric populations.

Lerna was excavated in the 1950's under the direction of John L. Caskey and the American School of Classical Studies in Athens. The excavation was conducted using a very high standard for the collection of human remains. Angel's study of the assemblage greatly assisted in my analysis (Angel 1971). All parts of the skeleton were present in the sample, which allowed for many sexing and ageing methods to be used. The completeness and proper storage of the assemblage suggests the demographic analysis from Lerna is acceptable.

4.6.4 SYRIA

Jerablus is a recent excavation using modern methods that have recovered a great deal of human skeletal material. The type of tombs and lack of post-mortem damage have allowed for much material to survive. The presence of foetuses in the assemblage also attests to this. Therefore taking into account this is an incomplete sample, as all excavations are, the demographic profile may be an accurate representation for an assemblage from this time and location.

CHAPTER 5

STATURE AND NON-METRICS

5.1 STATURE
5.1.1 INTRODUCTION

Stature has been interpreted as a variable with a strong genetic component related to climate adaptations as well being modified at the individual or population level by environmental factors, such as nutrition and health (Hernández et al. 1998). Stature will be used in this study as one more component in the overall comparison of the biological affinities of these samples. The stature of these samples will also be compared to other sites in the eastern Mediterranean.

The stature estimates from the human remains in this study are from very few limb bones. Some assemblages yielded many limb bones while others yielded none, such as Souskiou and Ayios Iakovos. Many anthropological reports combine all the limb bones to estimate the stature, and some do not mention which limb bones were used. Stature estimates can be made from any limb bones but estimates based on leg bones are more reliable because the leg bones make a direct contribution to stature, whereas the arms do not. For this reason upper and lower limbs of the stature estimation for males and females are presented separately in this section. Other than Lerna, there are very few limb bones from most of the sites. All the limb bones from Jerablus are from Tomb 302 except for one tibia from Tomb 2165. All of the stature estimates were determined from measurements taken by the author as discussed in the Method Chapter (3.7).

5.1.2 MALE STATURE

There were very few upper and lower limb bones to determine the male stature. The tallest average stature is from Jerablus at 172.92 cm and the next tallest is from Enkomi at 168.80 cm (Figure 5.1). The shortest statures are from Asine and Mosphilia, but since the number of limb bones is so small these figures are not very reliable. The males from Lerna are short and stocky even though it is an important and rich site in Greece (Angel 1972). Although the males from Lerna are short, they are still taller than the average for ancient Greek males (162-163 cm) (Angel 1946). Figure 5.1 helps to compare the average stature from each site.

5.1.3 FEMALE STATURE

Although there are few female limb bones there appears to be the same pattern present as with the male stature. Jerablus and Enkomi represent the tallest people from the samples (Figure 5.2). Lemba-Lakkous and Kissonerga-Mosphilia are similar in their statures while the stature from Lerna is slightly taller. As with the males, the females from Lerna are at the upper end of the average for ancient Greek females (153-154 cm) (Angel 1946).

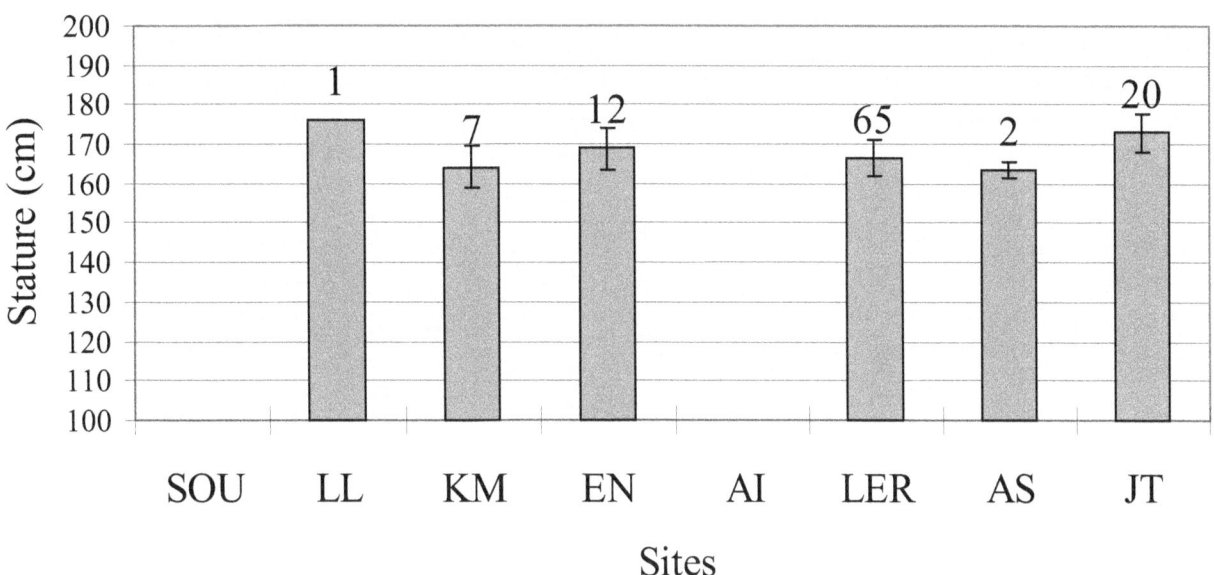

Figure 5.1 – Male average stature from combined long bones (With standard deviation and number of bones in each average).

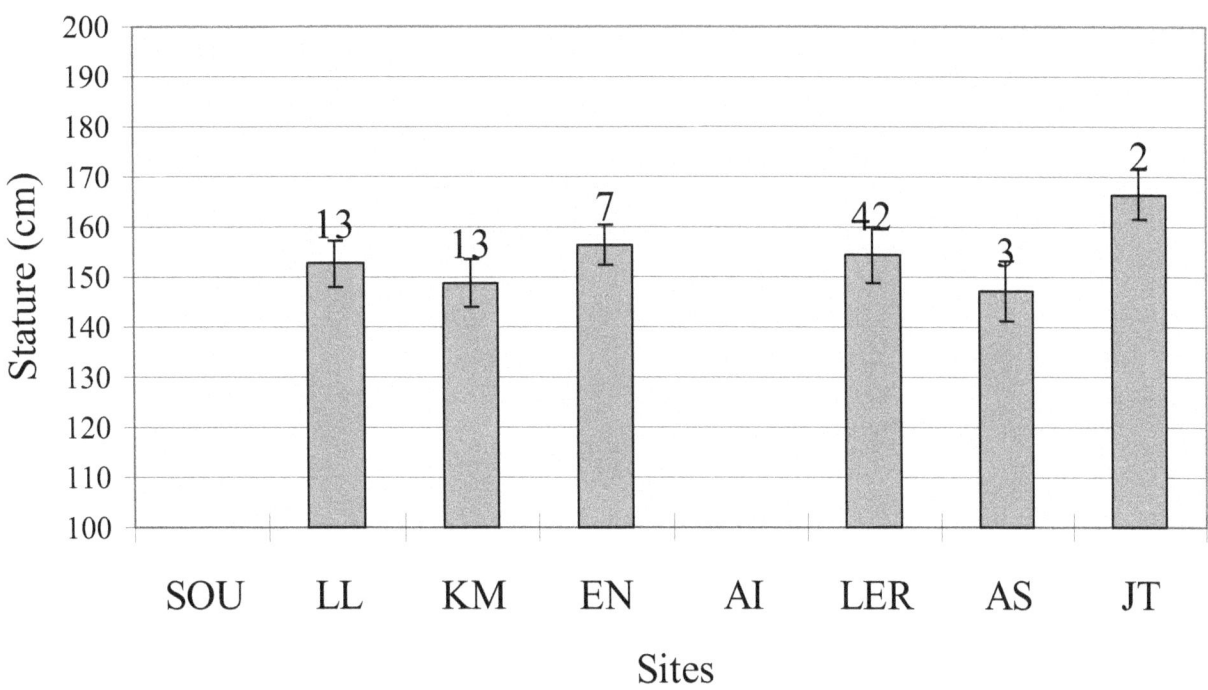

Figure 5.2 – Female average stature from combined long bones (With standard deviation and number of bones in each average).

5.1.4 COMBINED MALE AND FEMALE STATURE

Combining the male and female statures shows the same pattern as in the separate graphs. Averaging all of the stature figures and not simply averaging the male and female figures together calculated the combined averages. Jerablus and Enkomi have the tallest statures while Lemba-Lakkous and Kissonerga-Mosphilia have almost the same stature (Figure 5.3). Lerna has a taller stature and Asine (which has too few limb bones to give an acceptable stature) has the shortest of all the sites. Regarding Asine, Nordquist suggests the reduced height is due to a lack of meat protein and calories in the childhood diet (Nordquist 1987). This may be reflected in the above stature estimates. Most of the stature data comes from the upper limb bones, which usually suggests a taller estimate; in this case the stature is a short one.

Jerablus and Enkomi both have the tallest statures. Even though these sites are at opposite ends of the Bronze Age, they share some similarities. The first is most of the bones from Jerablus are mainly from the large chamber Tomb 302 and from Enkomi all the remains also come from large, well built chamber tombs. Compared to the statures from the other sites, which are lower, come from tombs, which are not as large or well constructed as Jerablus and Enkomi. The second similarity is both sites are rich in grave goods and were important centres in their regions. The taller stature has much to do with health and can be related to wealth and status. While the smaller settlements from southwest Cyprus have some of the shorter people, these differences have more to do with the wealth and health of the individuals buried.

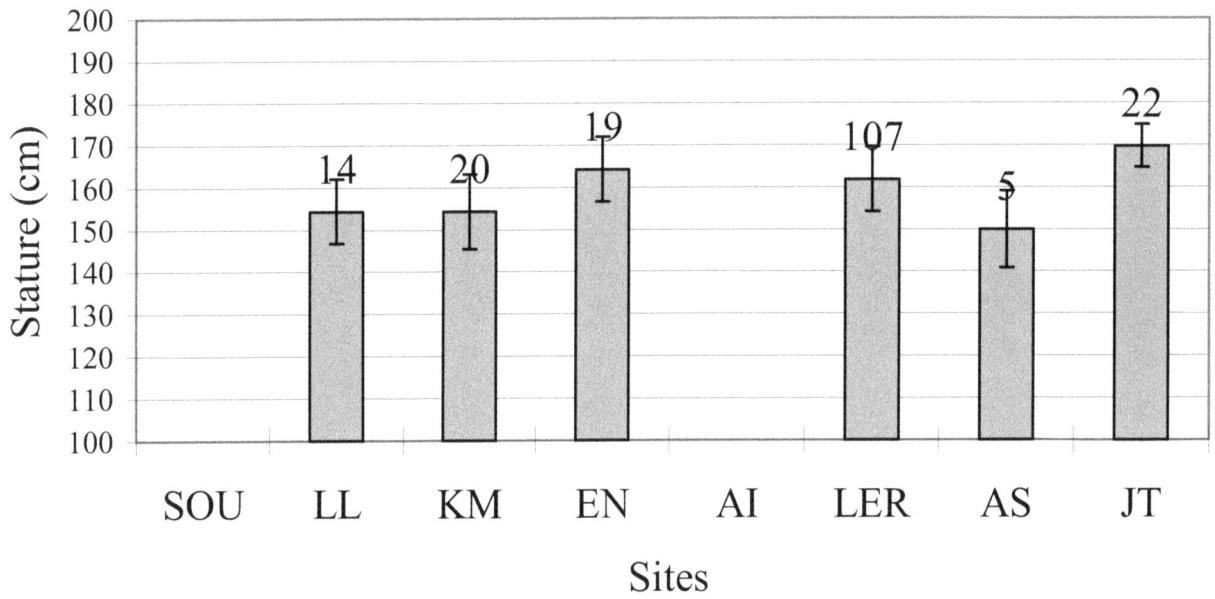

Figure 5.3 – Male and female average stature from all long bones (With standard deviation and number of bones in each average).

The males in this study fall within the range of stature from the study done by Formicola & Franceschi (1996) on stature estimation on Neolithic and Upper Palaeolithic peoples. Their range for Neolithic males is very short from 152.3 cm to very tall at 187.5 cm. Their study also determined a range for Mesolithic stature for females, between 150.3-155.7 cm. The samples in this study fall within the male range from the Neolithic, which is very broad. Unlike the female range, which is narrower, the samples in this study have a broader range.

5.1.5 REGIONAL STATURE COMPARISON

The sites in this study have been combined into various regions. Southwest Cyprus has the statures from Lemba-Lakkous and Kissonerga-Mosphilia. Northeast Cyprus only comprises Enkomi. Greece comprises Lerna and Asine while Syria has only the site of Jerablus. Comparing the regions in this study with other sites around the eastern Mediterranean, Jerablus still has the tallest stature (Table 5.1). The site closest to Jerablus is the Turkish site of Şeyh

Höyük, which is contemporary with the Tell Halaf culture of northern Mesopotamia and Syria (Şenyürek & Tunakan 1951; Şenyürek 1955). The site also corresponds approximately to the first half of the 4th millennium just as Jerablus. The combined stature from Şeyh Höyük is shorter for both males and females when compared to Jerablus (Table 5.1) (Şenyürek & Tunakan 1951). These remains were not excavated from a proper burial but from a refuse pit, making them quite different from the remains from Jerablus, which come from proper burials.

The late 3rd millennium site of İkiztepe in southern Turkey also has a smaller average stature than Şeyh Höyük and Jerablus (Becker 1988). These burials seem to be simple pits in a possible cemetery burial with only one being a pithos burial with few grave goods.

Sites	Males		Female		Combined		References
	Average	No.	Average	No.	Average	No.	
Şeyh Höyük	171.42	12	153.50	18	162.46	30	Şenyürek & Tunakan 1951
Karataş-Semayük	166.30	72	153.50	58	159.90	130	Angel 1970
İkiztepe	160.33	6	158.00	5	159.42	11	Becker 1988
Ayios Kosmas	-	-	149.00	4	149.00	4	Angel 1958
Keos	168.70	3	152.90	1	160.80	4	Fountalakis 1986
Manika-Chalkis	169.33	3	156.00	2	162.67	5	Angel 1977
SW CY	170.07	8	150.77	26	160.42	34	This Study
NE CY	168.80	12	156.40	7	162.60	19	This Study
GR	165.01	67	150.79	45	157.90	112	This Study
SY	172.92	20	166.50	3	169.71	23	This Study

Table 5.1 – Regional stature comparison (cm) (The number from Karataş-Semayük (Angel 1970) and Keos (Angel 1977) represent individuals and not limb bones).

Angel considers the stature from Karataş-Semayük as normal for this time period in the Near East (Angel 1970). It is clear the stature for Jerablus is higher than these figures, suggesting the stature for Jerablus is not an accurate representation of this site and time period. The difference in stature could have to do with the difference in health and status between the people buried in the more elaborate chamber tombs from Syria and the simpler burials from western Turkey. More limb bones need to be excavated to give a better overall representation of the stature from Jerablus.

The samples from Greece, Manika-Chalkis and Ayios Kosmas, are both on the mainland while Keos is on the Island of Kephala in the Cyclades. The samples from all of these sites are very small, which is the inherent problem with Aegean anthropology. Manika-Chalkis, which is Early Helladic, has a taller stature than the combined Greek sites (Lerna and Asine) (Fountalakis 1985). The combined Greek stature is lower with the inclusion of the low Asine stature, but the Manika-Chalkis stature is actually closer to the Lerna combined stature of 161.77 cm (No. 107). The stature from Ayios Kosmas, from the Early Helladic site in Attica, has the shortest stature in this comparison and should not be considered reliable because of the small sample size (Angel 1959). Keos is a Neolithic site but still falls within the range of Greek stature (Angel 1977).

There are also some fragments of human remains from Dendra in the Pelleponnese, with a stature for the few males, from tombs 13 and 14, ranging from 168 to 175.5 cm (Gejvall 1977). This stature estimate seems rather high compared to the estimates in Table 5.1, which range from 149 to 162 cm.

5.1.6 SUMMARY

It appears the tallest stature from Jerablus may not be reliable when compared to other sites in the region. Given the small sample of limb bones, coming mainly from one tomb, this also should be an indication of unreliable stature estimation for the entire population. The stature for the two sites in southwest Cyprus are very similar to each other, as well as being within the range of the Aegean and Anatolian sites (including northeast Cyprus). Lerna seems to have the same stature range as the other Greek sites in the region, while Asine with too small a sample size is not reliable. All of the sites with adequate sample sizes can be treated as reliable stature estimates.

5.2 CRANIAL AND POST CRANIAL NON-METRIC TRAITS

5.2.1 INTRODUCTION

Along with the dental non-metric traits collected in this study, cranial and post-cranial traits were also recorded. The frequencies for cranial traits are in Appendix 3 and the post-cranial frequencies are in Appendix 4. In other studies these traits would have also been used with the $D.\theta$ and the MMD statistics. Since the number of remains from these sites was limited, few of these traits were found. Therefore the data will be presented and not subjected to the same statistics as the teeth were. As already mentioned, there are so few traits from all the samples, traits were recorded from both sides and both sexes are combined in the frequencies.

5.2.2 CRANIAL NON-METRICS

Since there are very few data for the traits, the frequencies have been grouped by region. Northeast Cyprus has the highest frequency of ossicles at lambda, in the lambdoidal suture, ossicles at bregma and ossicles in the coronal suture (Figure 5.4). A high frequency of these traits can be associated with cranial deformation (Angel 1961; Ossenburg 1970; 1976). The practice of cranial deformation in Cyprus has been recorded from Neolithic Erimi and Khirokitia (Angel 1953). However there is no evidence of any cranial deformation from Neolithic Sotira (Angel 1961: Domurad 1986) just north of Kourion and in Neolithic to Middle Bronze Age skulls on the north coast (Buxton 1920; Hjortsjö 1947). There is also no evidence of any deformation from the sites in this study from southwest Cyprus. Even though no complete crania were found from these sites, ossicles and usually occur with this type of deformation are not present in the southwest region.

Out of 28 individuals examined from Ayios Iakovos, ten showed definite signs of cranial deformation, or 36% of the total population. Three children were also identified with signs of cranial deformation but since skeletal non-metric traits are only recorded in adults, only the adults will be considered in this study. Including the extra individuals from Fischer's report (Fischer 1986) the total proportion of individuals with cranial deformation is 25%. Out of the 59 adults examined from Enkomi, there are 46%, which exhibit cranial deformation. Including the extra specimens from Fischer's report, the total proportion of cranial deformations is 39%. Two children were also identified with signs of cranial deformation. This high incidence of cranial deformation from the northeast Cypriot sites helps to explain the high incidence of ossicles in the cranial sutures.

The sites with cranial deformation – Enkomi, Ayios Iakovos and Neolithic Khirokitia and Erimi – suggest this trend being one of custom rather than genetics, since it does not occur at Sotira or the southwest Cypriot sites. Without examining the remains from other sites in Cyprus it is difficult to determine the reason for this difference.

Although there is a frequency of 0.09 for ossicles in lambda from Greece and Syria, these seem to represent the normal representation of traits for these regions, since no signs of cranial deformation were observed. Angel also does not mention any signs of cranial deformation from Lerna, which he points out was rare in ancient Greece (Angel 1971).

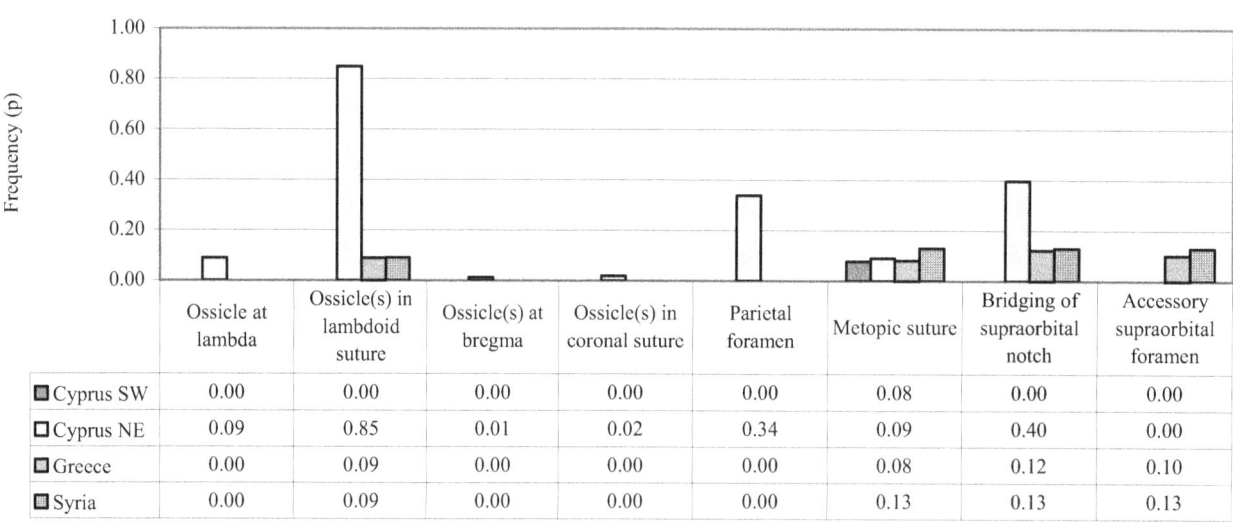

Figure 5.4 – **Cranial non-metric trait frequencies by region.**

From the graph it is evident there are very few cranial traits present for southwest Cyprus. The metopic suture is present with a frequency of 0.08 (No. 26), and the frequencies from northeast Cyprus and Greece are very close. Only Syria has a slightly higher frequency than the other sites. The metopic suture is one of the traits found in excess at Neolithic Khirokitia, where it affects 17% of the sample of 71, which is normal for Europeans (Torgersen 1951; Angel 1953). The Bronze Age cemetery in Kalavasos village, in the Vasilikos Valley in south central Cyprus, also has some incidence of metopism (Schulte-Campbell 1986). Ossicles in the lambdoidal suture as well as cranial deformation was also observed from Kalavasos.

The high frequency of the bridging of the supraorbital notch trait for northeast Cyprus may be due to the high proportion of cranial deformation. This trait is present in Greece and Syria but again in small frequencies and absent in southwest Cyprus. The accessory supraorbital foramen trait is only found in the Greek and Syrian samples and not in the Cypriot assemblage.

5.2.3 OTHER SAMPLES AROUND THE EASTERN MEDITERRANEAN

There have been many studies conducted on samples from around the world and there were many studies to choose from to compare to the samples in this study. There are none from any of the coutries where this study's samples are from.

Three samples included for comparison are from two Egyptian assemblages and one from the Levant. The Egyptian sample has 48 skulls from the pre-dynastic period of the Badari culture (c. 4400-4000 BC) (Morant 1935; Berry et al. 1967). The second is a sample of 55 skulls from dynasties XII-XVIII (1991-1300 BC) (Berry and Berry 1967). These two assemblages are close in time to the earlier Cypriot sites and with the Greek and Syrian sites. The final assemblage was a large sample of 54 skulls from the Iron Age site of Lachish (c. 700 BC) (Risdon 1939; Berry and Berry 1967). The site of Lachish is dated well after the Bronze Age but is still close, geographically and temporally, to the LBA Cypriot sites for an appropriate comparison. All data from the three sites have been combined by sex and by side (Berry 1979). Frequencies of these samples are in Appendix 7.

The northeast Cypriot sample has the lowest frequency of ossicles at lambda at 0.09, while the highest value is from Dynastic Egypt at 0.15, then Lachish, and Badari (Table 5.2). Again the northeast Cypriot sample seems to dominate the ossicles in lambda trait, with the Dynastic, Badari and Lachish traits all clustered between the values of 0.30 and 0.29 (Table 5.2). The ossicles at bregma trait, from the table, are self explanatory with only the northeast Cypriot site with the trait present. Lachish has the highest frequency at 0.037, with the ossicles in the coronal suture trait, but the values from the other samples are low and close together.

Traits	Dynastic Egypt	Badari	Lachish	SW Cyprus	NE Cyprus	Greece	Syria
Ossicle at lambda	0.15	0.10	0.11	-	0.09	-	-
Ossicle(s) in lambdoid suture	0.25	0.30	0.3	-	0.85	0.09	0.09
Ossicle(s) at bregma	-	-	-	-	0.01	-	-
Ossicle(s) in coronal suture	-	0.02	0.04	-	0.02	-	-
Parietal foramen	0.56	0.32	0.35	-	0.34	-	-
Metopic suture	0.04	0.06	0.07	0.07	0.09	0.08	0.13
Bridging of supraorbital notch	0.1	0.15	0.18	-	0.4	0.12	0.13
Accessory supraorbital foramen	0.39	0.18	0.19	-	0	0.10	0.13

Table 5.2 – Cranial non-metric trait frequencies by region.

The Parietal foramen is dominated by the dynastic sample with a frequency of 0.56 and Badari, Lachish and northeast Cyprus ranging between 0.32 and 0.35. The metopic suture shows all of the sites clustered between 0.062 from Badari and 0.13 from Syria. These metopic suture values are within the expected range for eastern Mediterranean populations (Berry 1968). The northeast Cypriot sites have the highest value for the bridging of the supraorbital notch, with a frequency of 0.4 while the rest of the sites (except for southwest Cyprus) range between 0.18 and 0.1. The Egyptian dynastic sample has the highest frequency of 0.39 for the accessory supraorbital foramen trait. The Badari and the Lachish samples are close, between 0.181 and 0.185 respectively. The Greek and Syrian samples are slightly lower at frequencies of 0.10 and 0.13 respectively.

5.2.4 SUMMARY

There is an obvious difference in lambdoid ossicle frequency between the sample from northeast Cyprus and the rest of the assemblage in this study. This most likely has to do with the high proportion of cranial deformation, which occurs in the region. The other sites do not differ greatly among the traits present.

The comparison with the other sites around the eastern Mediterranean shows northeast Cyprus does not seem to be the most distinctive group. Northeastern Cyprus has the highest frequency with only two traits, while dynastic Egypt has the highest frequencies with three traits.

Risdon makes reference to eight skulls from Lachish (out of 731), all from the same tomb, which show signs of cranial deformation (Risdon 1939). He is not sure whether the deformation is artificial or natural. Risdon also mentions a high proportion of ossicles in the coronal suture, as well many ossicles in the lambdoid suture. This suggests the high proportion of ossicles at lambda, in the lambdoid suture and in the coronal suture, are normal and not due to cranial deformation for Lachish (Table 5.2). Although it is unknown which skulls from the sample Berry and Berry included in their study, according to Risdon there is still a high frequency of ossicles in the skulls even though there are not very many identified deformed skulls (Risdon 1939).

The samples from Greece and Syria seem to be different from the Egyptian and Lachish samples, with similarities in three traits. Only with the metopic suture does the Syrian sample have the highest frequency but this may be due to a small sample size.

5.3 POST-CRANIAL NON-METRICS
5.3.1 INTRODUCTION

As with the cranial traits there were very few skeletal elements from which to record post-cranial traits. The main reason to present these data is for completeness in the documentation of all non-metric traits from these sites, and so other researchers can use these data in their non-metric studies. Unlike the numerous studies done on cranial traits, there are very few that deal with post-cranial traits. Therefore it will not be possible to compare these samples with traits from other sites. Perhaps in the future other studies focusing on post-cranial traits from the eastern Mediterranean will use the data presented here.

5.3.2 COMPARISON

From the sites in northeast Cyprus, only femora were present for study, therefore only the Poirier's facet and the plaque traits can be included in this comparison. All the sites, except for southwest Cyprus for the Poirier's facet trait, have a frequency between 0.41 and 0.46 with Greece having the highest (Table 5.3). Northeast Cyprus has the highest frequency of the plaque trait on the femoral neck. Both southwest Cyprus and Syria have the highest medial tibial squatting facet frequency while Greece's frequency is lower. The lateral squatting facet has similar frequencies between southwest Cyprus and Syria, which are close together, while Greece has a higher frequency.

Traits	SW Cyprus	NE Cyprus	Greece	Syria
Poirier's facet	-	0.41	0.46	0.42
Plaque	-	0.22	0.10	0.08
Medial tibial squatting facet	0.40	-	0.25	0.40
Lateral tibial squatting facet	0.40	-	0.72	0.47
Septal aperture	0.33	-	0.19	0.41
Vastus notch	0.07	-	0.18	0.21
Os trigonum	-	-	0.16	0.05
Medial talar facet	-	-	0.09	-
Lateral talar extension	0.05	-	-	0.05
Double inferior anterior talar facet	-	-	0.48	0.05
Double anterior calcaneal facet	0.25	-	0.53	0.17
Absent anterior calcaneal facet	-	-	0.05	0.06

Table 5.3 – Post-cranial non-metric trait frequencies by region.

The septal aperture trait found on the humerus again shows the frequency of southwest Cyprus and Syria being very similar, while the Greek frequency is lower. The vastus notch trait is more similar between Greece and Syria than to southwest Cyprus. The os trigonum trait only has frequencies for Greece and Syria.

The medial talar facet trait only has a value for Greece, while the lateral talar extension only has values for southwest Cyprus and Syria, and they are both the same. The double inferior anterior talar facet for Greece is much higher than the Syrian frequency. The double anterior calcaneal facet for Greece has a much higher frequency than southwest Cyprus or Syria. The absent anterior calcaneal facet has a similar frequency for Greece and for Syria.

5.4 SUMMARY

Not many conclusions can be reached given the available trait frequencies for northeast Cyprus. However there are four traits between southwest Cyprus and Syria, which have similar frequencies. These traits are the medial and lateral squatting facets, septal aperture and lateral talar extension traits. The Greek sample shares similarities with Syria on the vastus notch and absent anterior calcaneal facet traits. There is not much distinction between the Greek frequencies and the other regions.

CHAPTER 6

BIO-DISTANCE

6.1 INTRODUCTION

After recording the traits from the dentition, the frequencies were determined. Two equations were used to determine measure of divergence between the samples the Mean Measure of Divergence (MMD) and the Coefficient of θ ($D.\theta$). Most bio-distance studies usually include only the MMD equation. Therefore, by including both statistics in this study they act as a check against each other. The dental traits alone will be used in the bio-distance analysis between the sites. Cranial and post-cranial traits can also be used but the data from these samples are too small to be used with these equations.

Up to 35 morphological traits of the permanent dentition were included for this study, in accordance with the method and standards established by Turner et al. (1991). All the frequencies of traits observed are in Appendix 5. Only traits with ten or more teeth are included in the final analysis helping to eliminate small numbers of teeth, which would have affected the calculations (Nichol 1989; Johnson & Lovell 1994). The study by Johnson and Lovell (1994) only included back teeth in their MMD calculations because those teeth were available for study. This study includes teeth from all around the dental arcade.

Non-metric dental traits have ranges of expression and where the range might be from 0-6 for a single trait, only those traits that score 2-6, in this example, will be included in the analysis (Turner et al. 1991; Cucina et al. 1999). Therefore, traits scored 0-1 is considered absent (0) while 2-6 is considered present and are included in the analysis. This diminishes any observer error since any questionable trait data would not be included in the analysis.

Out of the maximum number of 35 traits as many as 23 traits were used, with some paired comparisons, and as few as two with others. Nichol (1989) suggests comparisons on less than 10 would result in less reliable comparisons, although the studies done by Scott and Turner in their sample of the Japanese used only 5 traits while their study on world samples used up to 9 traits (Scott & Turner 1997). Traits with less than 10 teeth present for any sample were excluded from the analysis. Therefore between two samples, if one had less than 10 teeth present that trait would be excluded from both samples in the comparison. The list of traits in Appendix 5 shows all teeth and traits recorded in this study. A visual inspection of the list shows which traits with less than 10 teeth were excluded. Although I have included some results with small numbers of traits, I believe these numbers can be helpful as a guide to biological relations between the samples. Some of the comparisons using less than 10 traits have positive MMD significance tests, which are considered valid. Each comparison has a different combination of traits in the calculations; this allows each pair to reflect its similarities and differences independent of the other sites, instead of having all the sites subject to the same traits.

Some traits were removed from the calculations, including the Metacone expression on M^1 and M^2 and the hypocone expression for M^1. These two traits almost always showed 100% presence. This was either due to recording error or to the inherent nature of the samples studied. Scott and Turner state that such traits: "…loses its status as a non-metric variant as it is present in all individuals."(Scott & Turner 1997:141). In order not to skew the calculations, these have been excluded from the analysis. With regards to the molar cusp pattern trait (Appendix 5), only the '+' pattern was included in the final analysis and not the 'Y' or 'X'.

6.1.1 MEAN MEASURE OF DIVERGENCE

The trait frequencies were determined using the Anscombe (1948) transformation for small samples and then the Mean Measure of Divergence (MMD) distance statistic was applied (Berry 1976; Irish 2000) (Appendix 8). The MMD was devised by C.A.B. Smith (Grewal 1962; Berry 1963), and modified according to the recommendation of Green and Suchey (1976) using the Freeman and Tukey angular transformation (Berry and Berry 1967; Sjøvold 1973; 1976-1977; Green and Suchey 1976; Ossenberg 1977). According to Irish, "This multivariate technique provides a quantitative estimate of biological divergence among samples based on the degree of phenetic similarity for all traits." (2000:398). It is assumed that phenetic similarity in dental morphology reflects the underlying genetic similarity (Irish 2000; Guatelli-Steinberg et al., 2001). A lower MMD value indicates greater similarity while a higher value indicates less similarity. This statistic assumes phenetic similarity and approximates cladistic relationship (Irish 1997; 2000).

The results from the MMD equation were also applied to a significance test recommended by Sjøvold (1973)(Ossenberg 1976; 1977)(Appendix 8). For the MMD to be significant at the 0.025 level, it must be equal to or greater than twice its standard deviation of the comparison (Irish 2000; Guatelli-Steinberg et al., 2001).

Once the traits to be excluded were determined for each paired comparison, the MMD analysis was carried out in the same manner each time. With so many comparisons to make between all of the samples, it would have been more complicated and more time consuming to have multiple comparisons for the data sets.

6.1.2 COEFFICIENT OF "θ"

A second statistic was used which determines the diversity coefficient "θ" ($D.\theta$) between two samples (Reynolds et al 1983; Tyrell and Chamberlain 1998) (Appendix 8). For this equation the Anscombe transformation was not used to determine frequency, instead the frequency was determined by simple arithmetic.

Tyrrell and Chamberlain (1998) used this equation in their study comparing the biological affinities between modern human populations and Neanderthals. They used a numerical analysis in order to determine a diversity coefficient similar to Wright's F_{ST} (Wright, 1951), which they have called the diversity coefficient "θ" (Reynolds et al., 1983; Tyrell & Chamberlain 1998). According to Reynolds (et al.): "...the coancestry coefficient is used as the basis for a measure of genetic distance for short-term evolution, when the divergence between populations with a common ancestral population may be regarded as being due solely to drift." (Reynolds et al., 1983:767).

This equation is useful because it is designed to measure the divergence between populations that is caused by genetic drift and by which mutation and all other forces affecting gene frequencies are excluded. This is also useful for smaller populations and where short-term evolution is expected (Reynolds et al., 1983).

The main difference between the two measurements of bio-distance is the MMD is based on the average difference in trait frequency between two groups, and the $D.\theta$ is based on the ratio of between-group to within-group variation in trait frequency. Therefore the $D.\theta$ can be regarded as a 'weighted' MMD, with the weights being inversely proportional to the within-group variation. The two measures therefore give similar but not identical results (Chamberlain pers. com. 2003).

As with the MMD analysis when the traits to be excluded were determined for each paired comparison, the $D.\theta$ analysis was carried out in the same manner each time. With so many comparisons to make between all of the samples, it would have been more complicated and more time consuming to have multiple comparisons for the data sets.

6.2 $D.\theta$ ANALYSIS

The first statistic used in biological comparison is the $D.\theta$ equation. The values represented in Table 6.1 are averages made up of all of the non-metric traits with each paired comparison. The comparison will follow a temporal progression from the oldest sites to the more recent, beginning with southwest Chalcolithic Cyprus.

All sites in southwest Cyprus are in close proximity and are contemporary (Appendix 1 - Chronology Table). It is immediately apparent that the closest sites, Lemba and Mosphilia, are not the most similar. They share a $D.\theta$ value of 0.914 while each of these sites is more similar to Souskiou, which is much further away. The implications of this will be addressed in Chapter 7 – Discussion. Since Souskiou is a looted cemetery it has a chronology based on ceramic dating and is not as reliable as the chronology from Mosphilia, which is based on reliable carbon dates (Peltenburg 1982b; Christou 1989; Peltenburg et al. 1998). Since the dating is not accurate, the relationship between Mosphilia and Souskiou (and the other sites) may have more to do with distance than time.

	SOU	LL	KM	JT	LER	AS	AI	EN
SOU		21	22.5	554	864	849	132	132
LL	0.790		1.5	546	850	849	148	146
KM	0.649	0.914		546	864	849	146	146
JT	0.663	0.750	0.882		1392	1377	417	384
LER	1.346	1.302	1.356	1.221		15	936	936
AS	0.822	0.542	0.701	0.618	1.258		924	921
AI	1.100	0.732	1.045	0.894	1.291	1.003		18
EN	0.662	0.731	0.698	0.695	0.747	1.543	1.189	

Table 6.1 – Pair-wise distances ($D.\theta$) between all sites. Upper part of matrix is geographic distances between sites.

Jerablus in Syria is contemporary with southwest Cyprus but are rather different culturally. In addition these sites are further away from each other and are separated by the sea. The sample from Jerablus seems to be more similar to Souskiou (0.663), than to Lemba or Mosphilia. This connection with the mainland and with one of the oldest sites on Cyprus may be an indication of a shared common ancestor. Comparing compared to Lemba (0.75) and Mosphilia (0.882) displays a similar closeness. This first series of comparisons show the closer sites geographically, does not necessarily make them the most similar biologically.

Comparing southwest Cyprus to Middle Bronze Age Greece, there is a shift in the pattern that has been observed. The comparison between Souskiou and Lerna (1.346) shows the second highest difference between two sites even though they do not share the greatest geographical distance. Jerablus and Lerna do share the greatest geographical distance (1,392 km) between each other while the $D.\theta$ is also quite high (1.221). The comparison between Lerna to Lemba (1.302) and Mosphilia (1.356) are also very dissimilar in accordance to their close geographical distance with Souskiou.

Comparing the results from Asine shows a mixed picture. The site's close geographic distance to Lerna produces a very high $D.\theta$ value (1.258), while Asine displays a much lower series of values with southwest Cyprus and Jerablus. Asine's small sample size may be affecting this analysis.

The final comparison is with Late Bronze Age Cyprus with the other sites. Enkomi and Ayios Iakovos are approximately 600 and 1100 years after the end of the time period of the Chalcolithic sites (Table 6.2). There is quite a difference between the results from Ayios Iakovos (1.1) and Enkomi (0.662) in comparison to Souskiou. Ayios Iakovos shows a strong relation to Lemba and Jerablus but less of one to Mosphilia and Greece. Enkomi shows dissimilarity with its neighbour (1.189) but a much closer similarity to Chalcolithic Cyprus. This difference between Enkomi and Ayios Iakovos is confusing and may be due to the small samples. It may also have to do with the demographic composition of these two samples. The evidence from the Demography chapter suggests these samples are under-represented in children and are not appropriate samples of the population, which may be misleading the analysis (4.5.3). The predominance of older adults and few children may skew the analysis because heavily worn adult teeth do not show as many traits as unworn teeth.

	SOU	LL	KM	JT	LER	AS	AI	EN
SOU		400	500	500	800	900	1100	1100
LL	0.790		100	100	400	500	700	700
KM	0.649	0.914		0	300	400	600	600
JT	0.663	0.750	0.882		300	400	600	600
LER	1.346	1.302	1.356	1.221		100	0	0
AS	0.822	0.542	0.701	0.618	1.258		0	100
AI	1.100	0.732	1.045	0.894	1.291	1.003		100
EN	0.662	0.731	0.698	0.695	0.747	1.543	1.189	

Table 6.2 – Pair-wise distances ($D.\theta$) between all sites. Upper part of matrix is rough approximation of temporal distances between sites.

Geographic distance is the main factor in this type of biological distance study, where the closer samples geographically are assumed to be more similar biologically (Rothhammer & Silva 1990). In this study time also seems to be an important factor in the analysis of these samples (Table 6.2). The sites that are closer in time may have separated from the common ancestor more recently, and therefore be biologically more similar.

Using the statistical computer software, Statistica™ (V. 4.3) a tree diagram was generated from the $D.\theta$ means (Figure 6.1). The diagram was generated using weighted pair-groups means and Euclidean distances. There seem to be two main groups where Lerna and Enkomi have been separated early on. Ayios Iakovos appears to be the next site to be distinguished from the main group, which is made up of Asine and has split off from two smaller grouped pairs of Jerablus with Lemba and then finally Souskiou and Mosphilia. The diagram appears to show the same close connection to southwest Cyprus and Jerablus while showing a closer connection to Asine than to the northeast Cypriot sites.

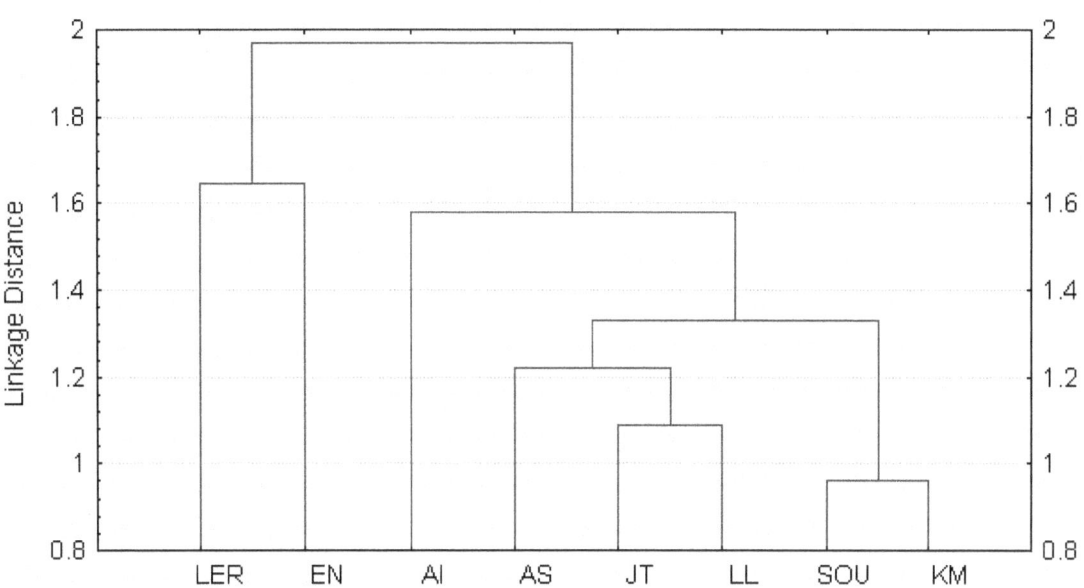

Figure 6.1 – Tree diagram of the $D.\theta$ means for all sites.

Time or geographical distance is not a factor in the tree diagram (cluster analysis) (Figure 6.1) and according to Derish and Sokal: "One would not expect hierarchic structure in human populations, especially at this scale, as they were never genetically isolated from one another, as species are." (Derish & Sokal 1988:822). Therefore these relations should be seen simply as relative to each other rather than populations joining or splitting. The cluster analysis method depicts the hierarchical pattern of similarity between the samples. It is effective insofar as the similarities really are hierarchical in nature. Data sets sometimes do not show a hierarchical pattern of similarity, and in such cases the clustering method is ineffective (Chamberlain pers. com. 2004). Scott and Dahlberg expand this discussion further:

> "Distance statistics, when used for inferring phylogeny, are based on the assumption that evolution is a branching process with the diverging populations showing constant rates of change through time. Genetic drift is assumed to be the primary mechanism generating diversity between groups because gene flow would result in the convergence of even distantly related populations, and depending on it's effects, natural selection would either impede or enhance the process of differentiation." (Scott and Dahlberg 1982:281)

The graph also displays the close relationship between the southwest Cypriot sites and Jerablus, and Lerna is the most different among the samples.

A three-dimensional scaling graph of the data was also generated using the program Statistica™ showing the relations between the sites (Figure 6.2). The use of Multidimensional Scaling (MDS) is a good method for visually representing relations between samples based on non-metric data (Safizadeh & McKenna 1996). The MDS method reduces the similarity or distance matrix to a smaller number of dimensions, typically three. This means the similarities/distances amongst n groups can be depicted in 3 rather than in n dimensions. This necessarily requires some distortion of the similarities/distances (to fit n dimensions into 3), however if most of the variation can be represented in the 3 dimensions then the representation will be fairly accurate. Unlike cluster analysis, MDS does not require the pattern of similarity to be hierarchical (Chamberlain pers. com. 2004).

Some observations from the MDS graph show Lerna separate from the main group and Jerablus is on the opposite end of the graph, which almost mirrors their geographic relationship to each other. It is also interesting to note that Asine is clearly clustered among the Cypriot sites even though its close geographical and temporal relationship is with Lerna.

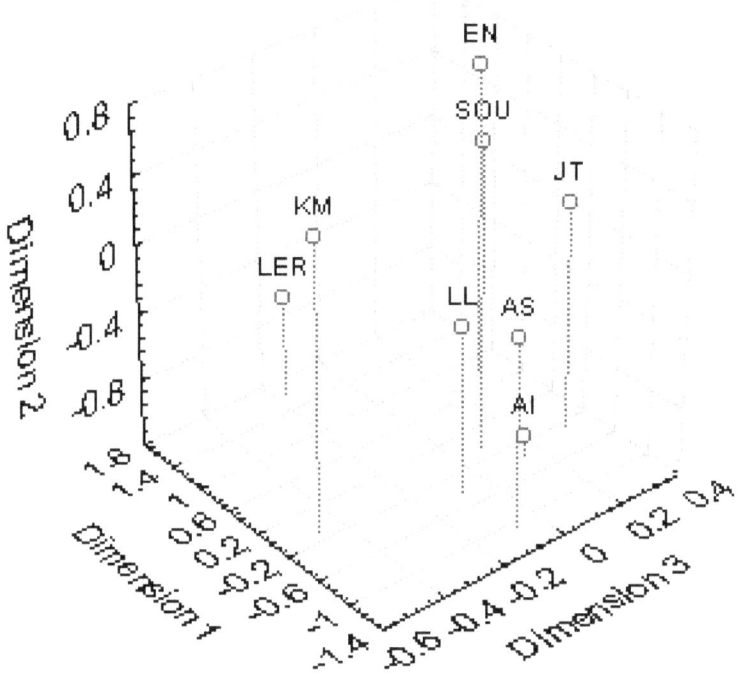

Figure 6.2 – Multi-dimensional scaling of the $D.\theta$ values from Table 6.1 (all sites)

6.2.1 SUMMARY

In summarising some of the patterns and trends observed in the $D.\theta$ averages, the sites of southwest Chalcolithic Cyprus all appear to be very similar as one would expect for sites in close geographical, cultural and temporal proximity. While the level of similarity between the 3 sites, relative to their distances, is not what one would expect with Souskiou clearly the furthest site with stronger similarities to Lemba and Mosphilia, which are closer to each other. There also seems to be an apparent connection between the Syrian site of Jerablus to western Cyprus. This could suggest a possible connection with Jerablus being part of the mainland parent population, which may have been responsible for settling parts or all of Cyprus. Without knowing more about other sites in Syria and in Anatolia, it is difficult to speculate about connections to a parent population. Lerna consistently was the most dissimilar site from the sample. This is what would be expected for the great difference in time and geographical distance from the eastern sites. Comparing Asine with Lerna, there is an unexpected dissimilarity between the two, given their close geographical, cultural and temporal relationship. This discrepancy may be due to sampling error from the smaller sample Asine.

It appears that in most cases the sites, which are the furthest in space and time, are not necessarily the most dissimilar. For example, Lerna and Jerablus share the greatest geographical distance but not the highest $D.\theta$ value. However Enkomi shows a greater similarity to Souskiou than to the contemporary nearby site of Ayios Iakovos.

6.3 MEAN MEASURE OF DIVERGENCE (MMD) ANALYSIS

The data in Table 6.3 represents the results from the second statistic used in this study to determine the biological affinities of the samples. Similar to the $D.\theta$ calculation, this second equation determines the Mean Measure of Divergence (MMD) between paired samples. This comparison is also ordered in same temporal progression from the oldest sites to the more recent, beginning with southwest Chalcolithic Cyprus.

Mosphilia and Lemba (0.062) have a strong similarity while Mosphilia and Souskiou (0.107) are less similar (Table 6.3).

Lemba's comparison to Souskiou has a negative MMD value and therefore is not significant. Comparing Jerablus to Mosphilia and Lemba displays a strong similarity between them, and the comparison with Souskiou is not significant.

	SOU	LL	KM	JT	LER	AS	AI	EN
SOU		21	22.5	554	864	849	132	132
LL	**-0.071**		1.5	546	840	849	148	146
KM	0.107	0.062		546	864	849	146	146
JT	0.043	0.133	0.152		1392	1377	417	384
LER	0.114	0.143	0.120	0.107		15	936	936
AS	**-0.066**	**0.027**	**0.102**	0.144	0.103		924	921
AI	0.345	0.206	0.136	**0.001**	0.204	**-0.128**		18
EN	**0.038**	0.203	0.136	**0.062**	0.071	**-0.038**	**0.009**	

Table 6.3 - Pair-wise distances (MMD) between all sites (Values in bold not significant). Upper part of matrix is geographic distances between sites.

Comparing southwest Cyprus to Middle Bronze Age Greece, Lerna shows some similarity with all the sites in southwest Cyprus and even more so with Jerablus. This is contrary to the results from the $D.\theta$ analysis where these two sites were the most dissimilar biologically as well as being the furthest apart in geographic distance. Lerna also shows a strong similarity to Enkomi. Asine shows some similarity with Jerablus and slightly more so with Lerna. Jerablus and Enkomi show some similarity but the MMD value is not significant (this sample almost passed the significance test).

Mosphilia and Asine show a figure that is not significant (this sample almost passed the significance test).

Comparing the results and the significance tests between Mosphilia and the Cypriot sites reveals a scenario of what one would expect. The comparison to Lerna is not what one would expect and the biological closeness of Asine can be disregarded given the small sample size from Asine. Jerablus displays a stronger similarity to Lerna than to Asine.

	SOU	LL	KM	JT	LER	AS	AI	EN
SOU		40	50	50	80	90	110	110
LL	-0.07		10	10	40	50	70	70
KM	0.10	0.06			30	40	60	60
JT	**0.04**	0.13	0.15		30	40	60	60
LER	0.11	0.14	0.12	**0.10**		10		
AS	-0.06	**0.02**	**0.10**	0.14	0.10			10
AI	0.34	0.20	0.13	**0.00**	0.20	-0.12		10
EN	**0.03**	0.20	0.13	**0.06**	0.07	-0.03	**0.00**	

Table 6.4 – Pair-wise distances (MMD) between all sites (Values in bold not significant). Upper part of matrix is rough approximation of temporal distances between sites.

6.3.1 SUMMARY

In summarising some of the patterns and trends observed in the MMD averages, the sites in southwest Cyprus do not show the same similarities, as do the $D.\theta$ values. The southwest Cypriot sites still share a clear biological connection, which is also reflected in time as well as geographical distance. Also the northeast sites share a clear connection with the southwest Cypriot sites. There is a definite pattern of relatedness between these 5 Cypriot sites, even though some values are not significant.

Using the computer software Statistica™, a tree diagram has been generated from the MMD means (Figure 6.3). The diagram was also generated using weighted pair-groups means and Euclidean distances. On the graph (Figure 6.3) Ayios Iakovos is the first site to split from the rest of the sites, the rest of the sites form 2 main groups. The first group comprises of Asine, Jerablus and Enkomi while the second group sub-divides the last four sites. Souskiou and Lemba form one group and Lerna and Mosphilia form the other.

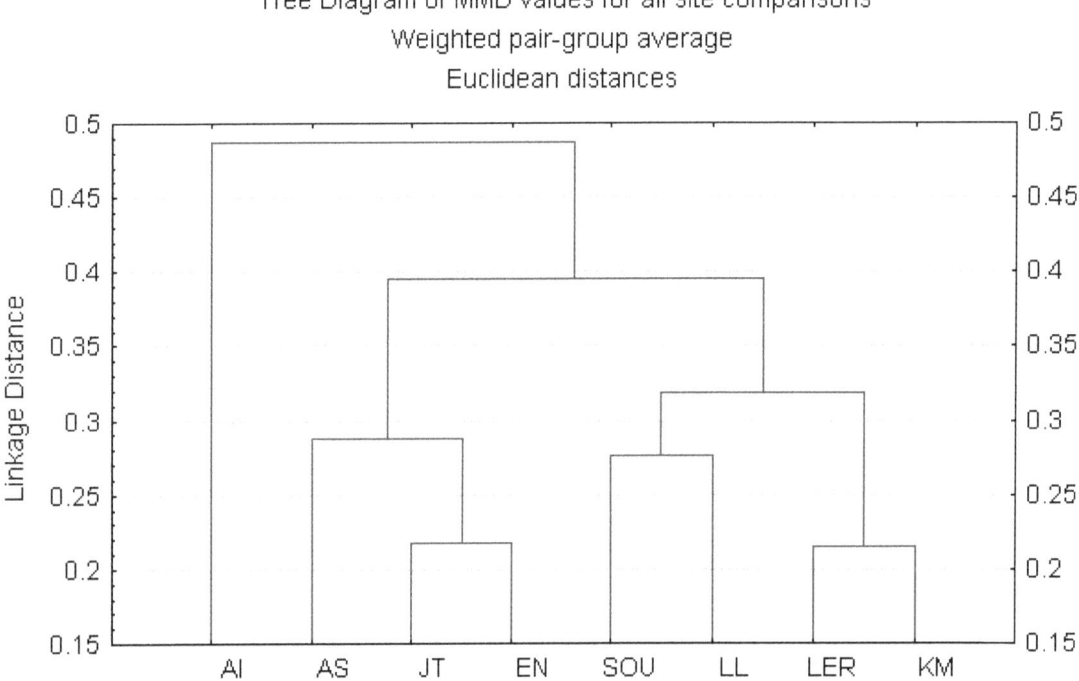

Figure 6.3 - Tree diagram of the MMD means for all sites.

As with the $D.\theta$ values, the graph shows a similar pattern with the grouping of the southwest Cypriot sites, with the added inclusion of Lerna, which is not similar to the $D.\theta$ results. In this comparison Jerablus is part of a separate group away from southwest Cyprus, which is grouped closer to Enkomi and Asine. A MDS graph of the data was generated using the program Statistica™ that also shows the relations between the sites (Figure 6.4). The sites from southwest Cyprus cluster together including Lerna (LER is hidden behind KM). While Jerablus is in the middle of all of the samples that suggest that it may have some common relationship with all of the samples in this study.

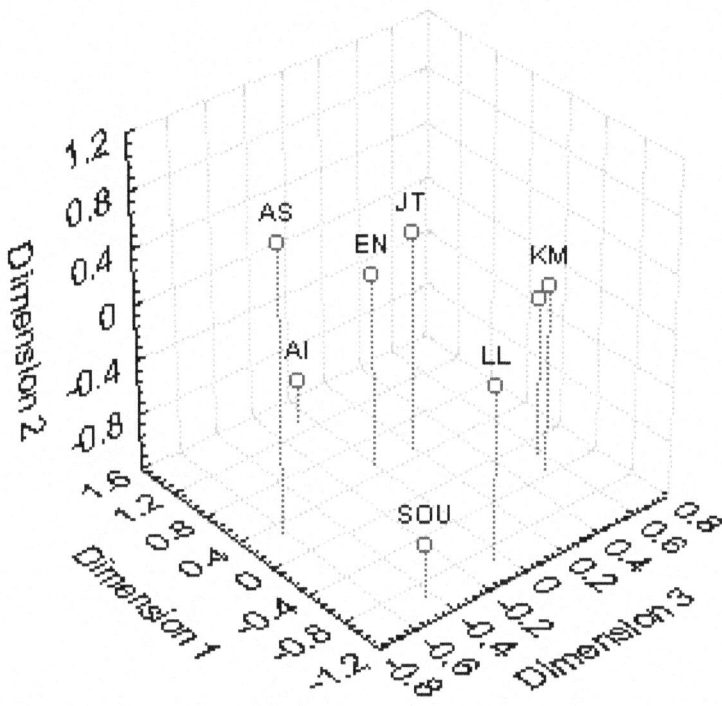

Figure 6.4 – Multi-dimensional scaling of the MMD values from Table 6.5 (all sites).

6.4 DISCUSSION OF THE $D.\theta$ AND THE MMD

After analysing all sites with the two statistics, there are some patterns present for both statistics. There is a definite relationship between the sites of southwest Cyprus, evident from the many comparisons as well as from the tree diagrams of the $D.\theta$ (Figure 6.1) and the MMD (Figure 6.3). The connection between Jerablus to the assemblage is mixed with the $D.\theta$ results suggesting a close connection to southwest Cyprus and the MMD results suggesting a connection to northeast Cyprus and Greece. These analyses cannot both be correct, therefore two possible conclusions can be reached are as follows:

i) The sample from Jerablus may have non-metric dental traits, which are common enough for the Near East and are shared by all of the sites.

ii) These comparisons do not take time into consideration; therefore the two different statistics may be amplifying the temporal differences between the sites.

These two conclusions will be addressed in the following Discussion chapter.

Northeast Cyprus shows a mixed relationship between all of the sites in the samples, and this is probably due to the small sample size from these two samples. This may also have to do with the cultural changes that took place in the eastern Mediterranean at the end of the Bronze Age and may be reflected in this analysis. The results from Greece are also mixed, with the $D.\theta$ showing Lerna to be distinct and Asine more similar to Cyprus, while the MMD results are the opposite. Excluding Asine, which is possibly an unreliable sample due to its small size, the different results for Lerna is puzzling. The two equations could be amplifying the differences between Lerna and the other sites, in the same way Jerablus may have been affected.

The way in which the two statistics deal with the given data may also be the reason for these differences. Both the MMD and $D.\theta$ generate meaningful biological distances between the samples and the discrepancies between some of the comparisons may be due to the possibility each is measuring different properties of the skeletal samples.

Another likely possibility is the two equations are reacting to differences between the samples. The MMD is a distance statistic based on the average difference in trait frequencies between populations, whereas the $D.\theta$ is a distance measure of the between-groups to total variation in trait frequencies.

Therefore $D.\theta$ can be viewed as a bio-distance measure that is weighted by the within-group variation in the samples. This means that it measures something slightly different from MMD. There are also differences that arise from the way in which MMD is calculated, in particular the subtraction of the so-called error term from MMD, which can lead to negative distances arising when populations are similar in trait frequencies (Chamberlain pers. com. 2004).

Another possibility is the data are homogenous relative to these statistics used and the differences observed are random low-level fluctuations. The $D.\theta$ statistic has only been used by Tyrrell and Chamberlain (2000) and has been shown to be useful when dealing with worldwide samples. It is unknown whether it is as effective at generating reliable bio-distances when dealing with samples that are much closer geographically and possibly, in this case, biologically. Therefore it is possible the MMD may be more useful for identifying differences between local populations (villages and towns). According to Turner (1992) MMD values from samples in Australia and Melanasia do not tie in closely to Asia but to African samples. He suggests this may be due to the differences in the way dental evolution works. Turner even speculates this may be evidence for the very great antiquity in Southeast Asia. However, this theory may not apply to my samples since they are much more closely related in time and space.

A similar dental study to determine the earliest inhabitants (colonists) of the Canary Islands revealed some inter-island MMD differences which are so slight that these differences may not be due to different founding populations but that "...isolation, genetic drift and the influence of local environments could have produced «some degree» of the morphological and genetic variation seen within the archipelago." (Guatelli-Steinberg et al., 2001:183). Regarding the MMD it is possible it may also have difficulty when dealing with closely related similar populations.

The cladistic representation of the different equations may make hierarchical connections where none exist in reality and add to the confusion of understanding the graph. According to Stringer and colleagues: "An underlying assumption of the cladistic method is that the samples are drawn from discrete populations, which are normally recognized species or higher taxonomic groupings." (Stringer et al 1997:391) Some of the problems with these assumptions regarding inter-species analysis is there is an unknown amount of gene flow between the populations and it is unknown whether there are ancestral samples within the living populations (Stringer et al 1997).

Using these two statistics together is part of understanding the way in which the samples relate to each other. Using only one equation, such as the more common MMD, would leave us with only one order of relationships for all the samples. By using two samples (in this case which do not concur) this raises more questions about the population relationships but also allows for an alternate interpretation. Since the data from these samples are studied for the first time, there is no way to know which equation is more accurate. The possibilities raised by using two equations allows for a broader discussion of not only the relationships but also in the way the traits are treated by the two equations.

6.5 COMPARISON TO OTHER SITES

Data from studies around the eastern Mediterranean have been collected from other scholars. As there are no published non-metric dental data of sites from the three countries in this study. In this comparison the sites in this study have been combined by time and region under the following abbreviations: Souskiou, Lemba and Mosphilia – SW CY (Southwest Cyprus); Ayios Iakovos and Enkomi – NE CY (Northeast Cyprus); Asine and Lerna – GR (Greece); Jerablus – SY (Syria). These samples will be compared to the following: a collection of northern Europeans from Reindeer Island, Lapps, Karilian Peninsula, Poundbury, Dorestad de Heul, Lent and the Danish Neolithic – EUR (Irish 1998; Stringer et al. 1997); a sample of Natufians, who are Mesolithic people from the Levant – NAT (Irish 2000); a sample of north Africans – NAF (Irish 1998); a sample of Early Bronze Age Italians – EBA (Cucina et al. 1999). The frequency data for each site is in Appendix 6.

6.5.1 THE $D.\theta$ COMPARISON WITH OTHER SITES

The $D.\theta$ means are presented in Table 6.5. Using the computer program Statistica™ a tree diagram has been generated from the $D.\theta$ means (Figure 6.5). The diagram was generated using weighted pair-groups means and Euclidean distances. Two main groups appear in the tree diagram. The first group contained the Natufian (NAT) sample, together with the north African (NAF) and Greek (GR) samples in a sub-group. The second group shows a split of the Early Bronze Age Italy (EBA) group. While the remaining cluster shows Syria (SY) split off from the remaining two Cypriot samples (NE CY and SW CY) along with the European sample (EUR).

	SW CY	NE CY	GR	SY	EUR	NAT	NAF	EBA
SW CY								
NE CY	1.136							
GR	1.291	1.204						
SY	1.224	0.919	1.527					
EUR	0.575	0.700	0.712	0.953				
NAT	1.141	1.491	1.179	2.159	1.230			
NAF	0.818	1.145	0.803	1.449	1.246	1.521		
EBA	1.637	1.386	1.704	0.910	1.561	2.461	2.592	

Table 6.5 – Pair-wise distances ($D.\theta$) between regions.

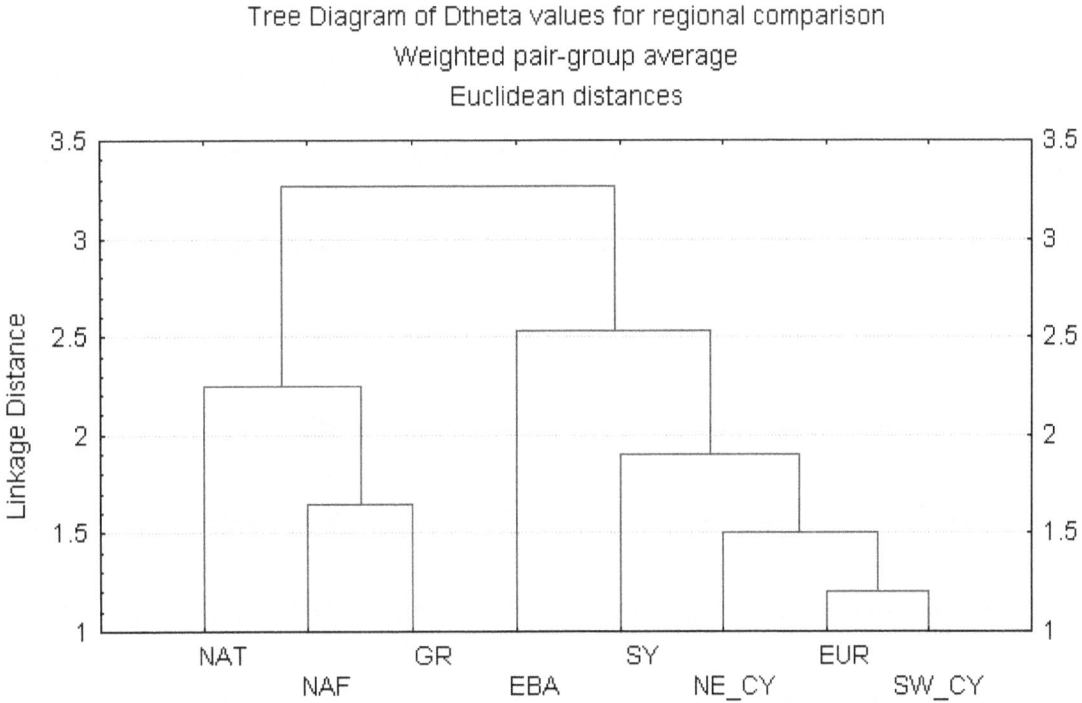

Figure 6.5 – Dendogram produced by mean linkage hierarchical clustering of the $D.\theta$ values from Table 6.4.

Within the two main clusters it is the oldest samples of the NAT (in the first cluster) and the EBA Italians (in the second cluster), which are the most different from the other groups. There is no connection between GR and EBA, which is interesting given their close proximity in time and space.

There is a close connection between the Cypriot samples and both the EUR average and SY, as was observed in the $D.\theta$ analysis above. A three-dimensional scaling graph of the data was generated using the program Statistica™ (Figure 6.6). The graph shows the similar site relationships as they appeared in the dendogram (Figure 6.5), with EBA, NAT and NAF on the fringes of the graph. The MDS graph adds an extra dimension to the analysis, which makes the relationships seen in the previous graph less straightforward.

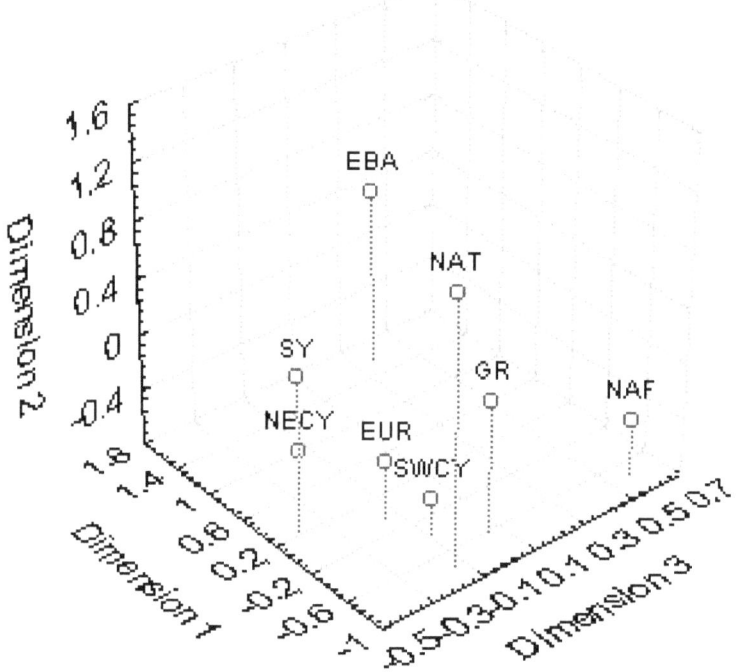

Figure 6.6 – Multi-dimensional scaling of the $D.\theta$ values from Table 6.5 (comparative sites)

6.5.2 THE MMD COMPARISON WITH OTHER SITES

The MMD means are presented in Table 6.6. Using Statistica™ a tree diagram has been generated from the MMD means (Figure 6.7). The diagram was generated using weighted pair-groups means and Euclidean distances. It is evident from the tree diagram that the NAT sample is the first to split from the rest. The next split shows EBA Italy and NE CY being distinct from the rest of the samples. The EUR and NAF samples show a strong relation, which may seem like an error. Other scholars have also seen this relationship between Europeans and Africans (Wijsmas and Neves 1986; Roler 1992). Irish (1998) and Stringer, who suggested that this similarity could be the result of gene flow (Stringer et al. 1997), also, noticed a similar relationship between Africa and Europe. The final grouping in the graph consists of SY, GR and SW CY.

A three-dimensional scaling graph of the data was generated which shows a mass grouping of most of the samples except for NAT and EBA, which are again on the fringes of the graph (Figure 6.8), just as they appeared in the $D.\theta$ analysis.

	SW CY	NE CY	GR	SY	EUR	NAT	NAF	EBA
SW CY								
NE CY	0.1531							
GR	0.1141	0.0473						
SY	0.1488	**0.0650**	0.1454					
EUR	0.2646	0.3029	0.3404	0.0812				
NAT	0.6992	1.3690	0.7111	0.4499	0.2724			
NAF	0.4146	0.4962	0.3599	0.1457	0.1147	0.1771		
EBA	0.6968	0.3037	0.5531	0.6044	0.4061	0.9386	0.4906	

Table 6.6 – Pair-wise distances (MMD) between regions. (Values in bold not significant).

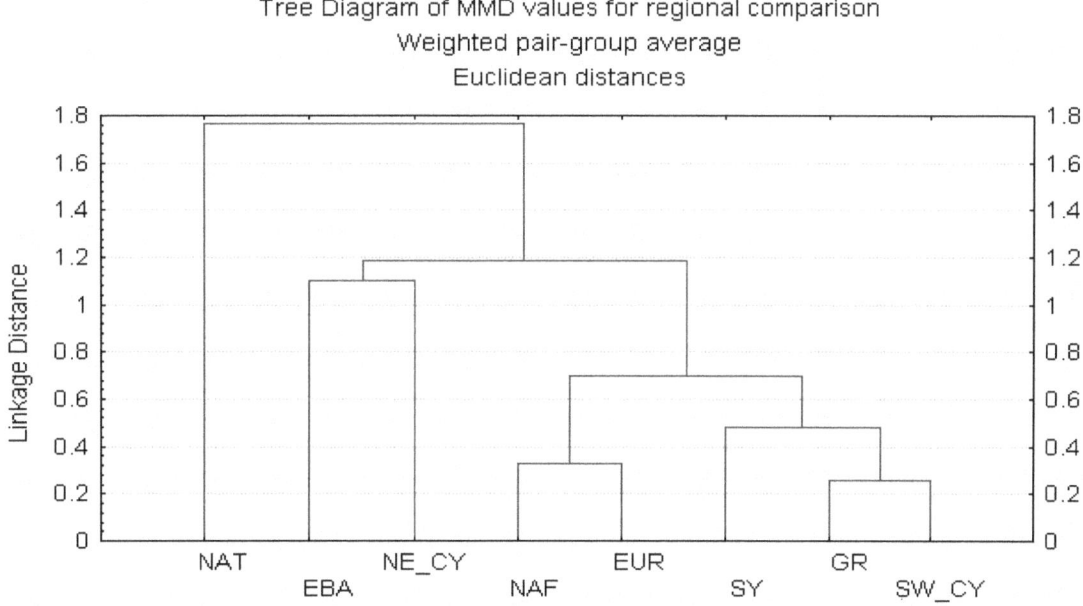

Figure 6.7 – Dendogram produced by mean linkage hierarchical clustering of the MMD values from Table 6.5.

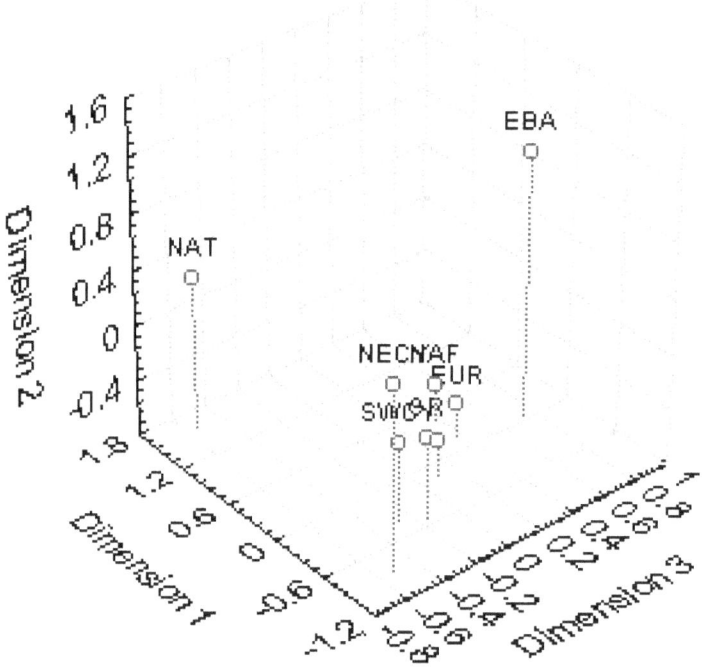

Figure 6.8 – Multi-dimensional scaling of the MMD values from Table 6.6 (comparative sites)

6.5.3 SUMMARY OF THE $D.\theta$ AND THE MMD REGIONAL COMPARISON

Using distance matrices should be taken with caution in regards to ancient populations where the evolutionary history is not known. Sometimes the distance matrix may show relationships, which cannot be explained (Scott and Dahlberg 1982). This may be the case with some of the results in this study. After analysing both statistics with these eight samples, there are some patterns that are present for both statistics:

1. There is a definite connection between the sites from southwest Cyprus to the Syrian sample, which is evident from the many comparisons conducted throughout this analysis.

2. The northeast Cypriot sample has a mixed picture between the $D.\theta$ and MMD. The $D.\theta$ tree diagram (Figure 6.5) shows a strong connection to southwest Cyprus while in the MMD analysis (Figure 6.7) it appears quite distinct from all the samples collected in this study. The small sample size and lack of teeth from the mandible may be affecting this analysis.

3. Greece also shows a mixed relation to the Cypriot and Syrian sites, but in both analyses it shows a clear distinction from the EBA Italian sample, which is interesting given their geographical proximity.

4. The Mesolithic Natufian sample is distinct in both analyses and also separate from the Syrian sample, which is interesting as they are close geographically but still separated by thousands of years. Suggesting that the Early Bronze Age Syrians are not descended from the Natufians.

The results from this analysis will be expanded upon in the following chapter. Archaeological and cultural evidence will be included in the discussion with the main focus revolving around the samples in this study and not the comparative samples.

CHAPTER 7

DISCUSSION

7.1. INTRODUCTION

This chapter will discuss how the data analysed in the previous chapters relate to the archaeological evidence in the eastern Mediterranean. This discussion will have two main focuses, Chalcolithic Cyprus and Late Bronze Age Cyprus, followed by a short section on artificial cranial deformation. Since the samples from Chalcolithic Cyprus are only from the southwestern area, for simplicity, when Chalcolithic Cyprus is mentioned, it is only the southwestern area that will be referred to. This study does not assume biological homogeneity of the entire island throughout the Chalcolithic from only three sites.

7.2.1. CHALCOLITHIC CYPRUS

The three sites in southwest Chalcolithic Cyprus are Souskiou, Lemba and Mosphilia. According to the analysis in Chapter 6, these three sites are closely related biologically which is expected, as they are very close geographically and temporally. In this case there is a correlation between biological and cultural relatedness. This should not come as a surprise, although having biological evidence to support this widely believed view is helpful. There are some differences between them that will be discussed below.

Addressing the question, are there any biological differences between the village sites (Lemba and Mosphilia) and the cemetery site (Souskiou)? The differences between these two types of sites have been discussed in section 2.2.6.1 and deal mainly with the location and treatment of the burials. Since Souskiou is the only Chalcolithic cemetery on Cyprus there appear to be some differences in burial practices from the more typical Erimi settlements. One of the differences is Souskiou is deficient in children and infants while having more adults than Lemba and Mosphilia (see section 4.2). This may due to different social practices between Souskiou (a cemetery) and Lemba and Mosphilia (settlements). At the settlements, people are buried under the houses of their family. In contrast, the burial practices at Souskiou show a different social custom, whereby a decision is made as to who is buried in the cemetery. According to the demographic analysis if people were being excluded from the cemetery population (infants and children) then it is probable to assume that certain people were included for social reasons. Peltenburg suggests Souskiou might represent a special burial ground for a regional population rather than simply for the adjacent village (pers. comm. E. Peltenburg 2003). If this speculation is correct then it may explain the demographic breakdown since it is not entirely inclusive. If there were a selection process involved in determining who is buried at the site, then this selection may have an affect on the dental non-metric analysis.

If Souskiou does represent a regional cemetery with a population made up of selected individuals from around the region (the size of the region is unknown), then it may be likely the biological affinities of Souskiou actually represent a much broader segment of southwest Cyprus. This theory does not imply that Souskiou contains people from Lemba or Mosphilia but that all these sites may share traits present in the greater population of southwest Cyprus. These smaller settlements, such as Lemba and Mosphilia, had their biological affinities affected by social, political and trade networks (Scott and Dahlberg 1982; Scott and Turner 1997). In this smaller scale there were differences between such local groups.

Even though there are differences between the MMD and $D.\theta$ equations one common thread is apparent. In the tree diagram of $D.\theta$, Figure 6.1, Souskiou is closely paired with Mosphilia and in the tree diagram of MMD, Figure 6.3, Souskiou is closely paired with Lemba (though not significant). In each case Souskiou is close to both sites but Lemba and Mosphilia are not as close to each other, contrary to expectation for two sites so close together geographically. This suggests Souskiou exhibits enough biological affinities from each site to be related to both. Lemba and Mosphilia share more traits between each other (23) in the MMD and $D.\theta$ analysis while the two sites share much fewer traits with Souskiou (8 and 7 traits respectively). Even though they share more traits with each other than they do with Souskiou, there is still a slightly stronger relationship between these sites and Souskiou.

The different demographic breakdown of these two types of sites may be reflected in the dental non-metric analysis and may have social implications. The unknown criteria of the selection process for the people being buried at Souskiou will affect the biological affinities of the sample. If the people from Souskiou are selected from a wide sample of the regional population then the biological affinities may show more generalities with other smaller samples that are village based, (like Lemba and Mosphilia) and where the locals are buried under the family houses. However, if the selection process for inclusion at Souskiou is determined on the social status of individuals (children as well as adults) the inclusion of some children may represent their importance through their familial relationship (ascribed status). Given the limited number of samples in this research it is unknown how this social interaction with the burial selection can realistically affect the biological affinities. The study of large samples from around Souskiou would allow for a more refined picture of the distribution of dental traits in southwest Cyprus. In addition the discovery of similar cemetery sites from the Chalcolithic period would also help to explain the complex social selection that is obviously occurring. For the moment Souskiou is a unique site during the Chalcolithic and any differences between settlement sites will generate more questions than answers regarding Cypriot burial customs.

The discussion of Chalcolithic Cyprus will also be in comparison to Jerablus and the biological similarities that are apparent from Chapter 6. Two possible theories for this relationship are: a) there is a long biological connection between Chalcolithic Cyprus and some of the more ancient colonists from the mainland, or b) there has been continuous contact with the mainland throughout the Neolithic and the early Chalcolithic. There is much evidence to support the first theory that people from the mainland colonised Cyprus (Stanley Price 1977a; 1977b; Todd 1986; Held 1992; Peltenburg et al. 2000a; 2001). There is less direct evidence for continuous contact between Cyprus and the mainland during the Chalcolithic. There is evidence for contact during the Neolithic, which diminishes over time and then reappears in the Early Bronze Age. This discussion will be based on the analysis of the: a) the anthropological and DNA evidence and b) the archaeological evidence.

7.2.2. ANTHROPOLOGICAL AND DNA EVIDENCE

According to the results from the MMD and $D.\theta$ comparisons, the sites from Chalcolithic southwest Cyprus all share similarities with Jerablus yet there are slight differences between them. This suggests proceeding further back in time the biological affinities increase between Cyprus and Syria (this may sound simplistic since the dating from Souskiou is not as reliable as from Lemba and Mosphilia, because is it mainly from pottery (Christou 1989)). This also suggests after an initial colonisation there was then genetic divergence on Cyprus. The MMD comparison shows the same pattern where the difference between Jerablus and Souskiou is not significant, but the other two sites fall in line with the distribution of sites by age. Since Jerablus is younger than Souskiou, this suggests they could share a common ancestor. This biological relationship with the mainland may also be a reflection of the type of traits present in the Near Eastern populations (close to Cyprus). In other words, this relationship may represent an ancient connection with the mainland that has not changed significantly over thousands of years. This also assumes there has been little extra biological influence on the mainland sample. These ideas will be expanded upon below.

According to current DNA studies, there is evidence for a wide reaching Neolithic migration across Europe, from the Near East, which occurred around 7,000 to 10,000 years ago (Cavalli-Sforza & Cavalli-Sforza 1995; Francalacci et al. 1996; Chikhi et al. 1998; Casalotti et al. 1999). In contrast, Mitochondrial DNA (mtDNA) studies suggest modern European populations are mostly made up of indigenous people who were in Europe since the Paleolithic (Richards et al. 1996; González et al. 2003). While these two theories agree there was a migration of people from the Near East in the Neolithic, the majority of current European mtDNA is not from the Near East. The earliest evidence for human occupation of Cyprus is no earlier than the Neolithic, therefore it is possible this movement of people from the Near East is represented in the Chalcolithic samples. According to dental studies by Scott & Turner (1997), all of the samples in this study should belong to the European group of world populations.

One reason to accept such continuity from the Neolithic to the Chalcolithic in Cyprus is the longevity of dental traits (Turner 1986). According to the studies carried out by Turner and his colleagues over the past 30 years on dental trait frequencies, for every 1000 years there is a change in the MMD of 0.01003 ± 0.004 (Turner 1985; Turner 1986; Turner 1992; Scott and Turner 1997). This number is very small and the greatest temporal difference between any of my samples is no more than 3000 years; this affects the MMD comparison in the present study very little. Based on this figure, the amount of 'normal' evolution (or change) is very small and may not be responsible for the degree of difference between the samples. Different environments can also affect the biological affinities of populations. The fact these samples occupy very similar environments rules out this factor as having a great effect on them (Rothhammer & Silva 1990). Therefore if 'normal' evolution and different environments can be ruled out in explaining the bio-distance data between these sites then the reason could be divergence due to genetic drift and the founder effect (Turner 1986; Scott & Turner 1997). Turner sums up this sentiment with the following statement: "How dental microevolution occurs is not clear, but it is seemingly quite regular." (Turner 1986:1142)

To illustrate the longevity of dental non-metric traits, a study conducted by Turner and his colleagues will be briefly explained. Turner and colleagues have extensively studied the people of Asia and surrounding regions. One study was on the people of Japan, which focused on two indigenous groups, the Ainu (who live mainly in the northern islands) and the main southern Japanese inhabitants. They compiled non-metric dental data of modern people from both groups and samples from modern day mainland China. They also included a limited archaeological sample of data from 3000 year old Jomonese and Chinese. From these samples they learned the modern day Ainu are more closely related to the ancient Jomon people and the modern Japanese are more closely related to the Chinese (Turner 1976; Turner 1979; Scott & Turner 1997). Archaeological and linguistic evidence suggests these conclusions are in agreement with archaeological as well as cranial and dental studies (Scott & Turner 1997).

After approximately 3000 years there is still a dental non-metric distinction between the Jomon/Ainu and Japanese/Chinese. In comparison, relating people from the Syrian Neolithic to the Cypriot Chalcolithic is also plausible given the same time span. This longevity may be because the Japanese islands act as a genetic barrier to insulate the people from external influence just as Cyprus may have done.

Another example of the longevity of dental traits of an isolated population is the study by Scott and Alexandersen (1992) on the Greenland Norsemen from 1000 to 1500 AD. Throughout that time period, the population became relatively isolated from Europe biologically. They experienced a change of climate with the mini Ice Age, and also had some biological intermixing with the Inuit who arrived after the Norsemen had established their settlements (Scott and Alexandersen 1992). In comparing the Greenlanders to Norwegians, there is evidence for divergence that may indicate the action of both founder effect and genetic drift. As it was known from where the Greenlanders had migrated, comparing them to European populations was an easy task. Due to the change in climate and diet, there was the added problem of determining whether differences found were the result of environmental or genetic factors (Scott and Alexandersen 1992:483). Scott and Alexandersen sum up their findings as follows:

> "In the context of their 500 year history which was characterized by marked changes in climate, fluctuating sociopolitical conditions, increasing isolation from the rest of Europe, and significant trends in a number of biological parameters, the most remarkable aspect of the Greenlandic dentition is its morphological conservatism. Despite changes in almost every other aspect of their life, their dental morphology maintained its fundamental European heritage to the end." (Scott and Alexandersen 1992:486).

The span of time Scott and Alexandersen dealt with is much smaller than the present study, but the changing climatic and dietary conditions affecting the Greenlanders are absent from my samples (Konigsberg 2000). This example helps to underline the longevity and stability of dental non-metric traits.

If Scott and Alexandersen had to compare the Greenlanders to samples all over Europe, they would have been more uncertain as to the level of similarities and differences between them. This is the situation with this study. The Cypriots may have come from Anatolia or Syria/Levant or both. If these samples from Chalcolithic Cyprus were compared to a sample from Neolithic Anatolia, perhaps they would exhibit more similarity than to the Syrian sample – or possibly the same similarity. Since these two possible parent populations are so close geographically, there are bound to be similarities and overlap in trait frequencies between them. This in turn suggests there may be close similarities between both and Cyprus.

Large populations are usually more diverse dentally, while smaller populations splitting off tend to become more specialised (Coruccini 1972; Scott and Dahlberg 1982; Schliwa et al. 1983: Scott & Turner 1997). This may be the reason for some of the results from Chalcolithic Cyprus. The $D.\theta$ of Mosphilia shows Souskiou is more similar even though Lemba is closer in time and space. The same situation is present in Table 6.1, where Lemba is closer biologically to Souskiou than Mosphilia, for the same reasons. Relative to the other sites in the study, the Chalcolithic sites are the most similar to each other but there are slight differences based on the splitting from the parent population and the specialisation that occurred (Coruccini 1972; Scott and Dahlberg 1982). All samples will continue to show similarities with the parent population but differences between them will occur determined by regionalism and/or social customs. This pattern, which Coruccini identified in studies done on southwestern Native North Americans, can be related to Chalcolithic Cyprus:

> "They formed a unified group when compared with several non-Southwestern skeletal samples. Significant genetic variability, however exists between each pair of populations, contradicting the idea of their belonging to a unified Pueblo Indian gene pool or to a fixed physical type." (Coruccini 1972:373).

The local populations will have organised themselves along social, political and trade networks and it will be these relationships, which will also dictate their biological exchange (Scott and Dahlberg 1982; Scott and Turner 1997). The daughter population does not require much gene flow to incur differences (Eller 1999), but genetic drift can be used to explain these differences (Coruccini 1972). Studies conducted on MtDNA have also shown that within major geographic groupings of humans there is a very low level of genetic variation. In contrast, however, these same studies find a much higher level of variation between groups (Relethford 1994). This corresponds with the dental non-metric results in this study.

Since all of these sites are in southwestern Cyprus we can only assume the sites further away will exhibit more divergence. The MMD analysis shows a similar picture but in two cases (Table 6.3) the figures from Souskiou are not significant and therefore not reliable. However, from the graph (Figure 6.3) the close relation between Mosphilia and Lemba is evident.

According to models in Scott and Turner (1997) the samples from southwest Cyprus represent the lowest level of differentiation – the village level. Making distinctions between local populations (villages) is difficult, as there are no standards for assessing biological distance between such groups (Scott & Turner 1997). Scott and Dahlberg add to this discussion with the following statement:

> "The rate of gene flow between any two sub-populations can be influenced by a variety of sociocultural factors and also by geographical distance. The interplay of marriage rules and distance essentially precludes random mating within a tribal population. Because of this, genetic drift will generate diversity among subpopulations;" (Scott and Dahlberg 1982:260).

Also, depending on the population involved in a particular study, differences between samples at the village level may or may not be present (Scott and Dahlberg 1982; Haydenbilt 1996; Scott & Turner 1997). This explains the differences between Lemba and Mosphilia. They are part of the same cultural group (Erimi Culture) but are slightly different biologically because they are sub-populations of the whole. Whether that whole includes all of Cyprus or just southwest Cyprus is still unknown. One must remember, however, when using skeletal analysis for historical reconstruction, the samples represent lineages and not biological populations (Ossenberg 1977).

7.2.3. SUMMARY

The evidence presented above proves this non-metric analysis is consistent with other studies indicating a splitting of a parent population. The local populations also show distinctions between themselves as well as connections to the parent population. The stability and longevity of dental non-metric traits suggest the parent population may be much older than the age of the samples from Chalcolithic Cyprus and Early Bronze Age Syria. This analysis does not suggest when this contact began and when it ended.

7.3. THE ARCHAEOLOGICAL EVIDENCE

The archaeological evidence favours Syria/Levant as a source for the Cypriot cultures rather than Anatolia, although this research has only one sample from Syria in which to make this connection. Therefore this research cannot endorse one probable location over another from only one mainland sample. Since there is an unsurprising biological connection between Cyprus and the mainland, it is important that an archaeological (cultural) connection also be made with the mainland. There is no other dental non-metric data from Syria or Anatolia to compare to the findings in this study therefore this limited evidence must be used with caution. There is very little direct cultural similarity between the Chalcolithic sites in Cyprus and Early Bronze Age Jerablus; the relationship therefore, must be a more ancient one, which could have its origins as far back as the Neolithic.

7.3.1. EARLIEST CONNECTIONS WITH THE MAINLAND

The earliest archaeological evidence suggests the first major cultural connection with the mainland was before the Neolithic. An early group of hunters had a small hunting campsite at Akrotiri (Aektokremnos) in the southwestern part of the island in the 11th millennium (Simmons 1991; Reese 1996). This settlement may have been temporary and did not produce a continuous human presence on Cyprus. There is recent evidence the first permanent humans to the island arrived in the 10th millennium B.C. This evidence also suggests that people arrived with domesticated plants and animals (sheep, goat, cattle, fallow deer, pigs, dogs and cats) (Ducos 2000; Peltenburg et al. 2000a; Vigne et al. 2000a; Vigne et al, 2000b; Peltenburg et al. 2001). This evidence comes from a number of sites around the island (Kissonerga-Mylouthkia, Parakklisha-Shillourokambos, Kalavasos-Tenta, Ayia Varvara-Asprokremnos and Akanthou-Arkosyko) (Peltenburg et al. 2000a; Peltenburg et al. 2001). The later Khirokitia (7th millennium B.C.) culture seemed to have evolved out of these earlier settlements with clear cultural connections to the mainland (Held 1992). According to Held, "...the Khirokitia Culture is an island-wide and culturally uniform phenomenon attested as a rule by open-air sites...fully sedentary village communities engaged in mixed farming and herding as well as hunting" (Held 1992:120). The cultural similarities between Cyprus and the Neolithic mainland that will be discussed are:

7.3.1.1. Subsistence Pattern
7.3.1.2. Artefacts
7.3.1.3. Burials
7.3.1.4. Houses and Architecture

The greatest similarity between Cyprus and the mainland seems to be with the earliest settlements of Kissonerga-Mylouthkia (hereafter Mylouthkia), Parakklisha-Shillourokambos (hereafter Shillourokambos) (10th millennium B.C.) and the later Khirokitia culture (6th millennium B.C.)(Mellaart 1965; Stanley Price 1977b; Peltenburg 1978; Peltenburg et al. 2000a; Peltenburg et al. 2001). There are many direct connections between 10th millennium Cyprus and the mainland while by the 6th millennium Cyprus had adapted the original culture to suit the constraints of an island existence (Peltenburg et al. 2000a; Peltenburg et al. 2001). By the 6th millennium, Anatolia and the Levant had moved on to other customs while on Cyprus they were practicing 7th millennium mainland customs (Stanley Price 1977a; 1977b; Peltenburg et al. 2001). According to Simmons (1994:1): "...there are few sociocultural antecedents with the mainland to explain Neolithic Cyprus." Even though the initial Cypriot culture came from the mainland, Neolithic Cypriot culture was local in character (Georgiou 1979).

7.3.1.1 SUBSISTENCE PATTERN

From the site of Shillourokambos there is evidence for the deliberate importing of domesticated pigs, sheep, goats, cattle, and with wild fallow deer (Stanley Price 1977a; 1977b; Held 1992; Ducos 2000; Vigne et al. 2000a; 2000b). Since there are not any wild ancestors of these animals, they were purposefully brought to Cyprus (Vigne et al. 2000a). The oldest caprines have been found in Tarsus (southeastern Anatolia), more evidence these first settlers came from western Syria and the Amuq region (Vigne et al. 2000a). Also the Mesopotamian fallow deer (*Dama mesopotamica*) comes from the Euphrates Valley again suggesting Syria as a more likely region of origin (Vigne et al. 2000a; 2000b). The fallow deer would become a main staple of the diet, more so than sheep and goats on the mainland (Croft 1985; Held 1992).

Since the domesticated crops of einkorn and emmer lack any antecedents on Cyprus, which also supports the idea that these crops were brought by Near Eastern groups (Peltenburg et al. 2001). The subsistence pattern from Khirokitia is also comparable to the mainland.

7.3.1.2. ARTEFACTS

The stone tools from Mylouthkia, bear similar pattern of retouch, from the Syrian early PPNB and from Shillourokambos and there is similar retouch from Byblos and Amuq points (Peltenburg et al. 2000b; Vigne et al. 2000a). By the late PPNB on Cyprus the Byblos and Amuq points show similarities as on the mainland (Peltenburg et al. 2000b). Peltenburg and colleagues suggest the term Cyprio-Pre-Pottery Neolithic B for this newly discovered period on Cyprus (Peltenburg et al. 2000b).

Certain features of the stone tool tradition first identified from Tell Mureybet on the middle Euphrates, have long been regarded as highly diagnostic of the PPNB culture in the Levant (Peltenburg et al. 2001). According to Peltenburg: "By about 9200 BP, this lithic package (Big Arrowhead Industries) had appeared in southeast Anatolia, the south Levant, and now Cyprus." (Peltenburg et al. 2001:49). Now these same lithic assemblages are being found on Cyprus, which clearly suggests it originated from southwest Asia (Peltenburg et al. 2000b).

The utilisation of obsidian appears to be typical of the Cypro-early PPNB (Peltenburg et al. 2001). During the Cypro-late PPNB changes to the lithic assemblage appeared, which may be more related to the realities of island culture, rather than to the isolation of the population (Peltenburg et al. 2001).

One example of a commonly traded commodity during the Neolithic and other times is obsidian. There is a much greater quantity of obsidian from Anatolia from the sites during the Cyprio-PPNB than from later Preceramic Neolithic sites (Vigne et al. 2000). Thirty-two obsidian blades have been found at the Neolithic site of Tenta that might have come from the Çiftlik source of south central Anatolia with some obsidian also found at Khirokitia, Troulli and Cape Andreas (Todd 1986; Åström 1989). According to Todd, "While such a quantity of obsidian does not indicate very extensive foreign contacts, the regularity with which obsidian blades occur throughout deposits of the Aceramic does suggest a steady supply which lasted for a considerable period of time." (Todd 1986:16). According to Mellink (1989; 1992), there has been an established trade route from Çiftlik through Cilicia since Neolithic times:

> "Cilician trade was already functioning as a middleman carrying obsidian from the South Anatolian plateau to the Levant, presumably from the aceramic period on. This suggests that the route through the Taurus Mountains (Cilician Gates) was seasonally functioning in the 7th millennium B.C.; early trade routes were beginning to develop linking the resources in the Acıgöl-Çiftlik area to a chain of sites extending to the Levant." (Mellink 1989:319)

The sites in northern Syria clearly fall within this area, that the people who later settled Jerablus may have been part of. Mountains and other geographic barriers traditionally have been thought to be genetic barriers between populations. A dental non-metric study conducted on Iron Age Italians, from both sides of the Apennine mountain range, discovered that time rather than geography had a greater impact on the biological affinities of the people (Coppa et al. 1998). In comparison, the Tarsus mountain range may have not acted as a barrier to gene flow between the region of Cilicia and northern Syria. The Cypriot evidence does not seem to conform to standard trading models (Todd 1986). Todd even suggests the obsidian may have come from a more indirect route, not from Mersin in Anatolia, but from Syria-Palestine (Todd 1986).

7.3.1.3. BURIALS

There is evidence of treatment of human remains from Shillourokambos and Mylouthkia, which are similar to ones observed in southwest Asia (Peltenburg et al. 2000b; 2001). Skull caching which was practiced in the Levant and southeast Anatolia seems also to have been transferred to Cyprus during the 10th and 9th millennium B.C. (Peltenburg et al. 2001). The burials from both of these sites are secondary burials, not primary. Therefore any direct comparison to the mainland from these (isolated) events should be treated with caution (Peltenburg et al. 2001).

The burial practices at Khirokitia are a mix of mainland traditions from late 7th millennium (Stanley Price 1977a). The practice of burying the dead under the floors of the houses (practiced at Khirokitia) was found at Çatal Hüyük (the only method used there), as well as at Jericho, which is older than the Neolithic site of Tenta (southeastern Cyprus) (Todd 1986; Åström 1989). Tenta as well as Jericho do not seem to rigidly adhere to the custom of burials under the houses. Some have been found outside structures, also practiced at various sites in Syria-Palestine (Todd 1986). As well, the use of red ocher to decorate the body is very common on the mainland but unknown on Cyprus (Todd 1989).

Another link with Syria/Levant and Khirokitia (and Neolithic Cyprus) is the lack of evidence of cranial deformation from Çatal Hüyük (out of a sample of over 200 burials) but was very prominent at Khirokitia (Angel 1971b; Domurad 1986; 1989). There was however evidence of artificial cranial deformation from Neolithic Jericho (Levant) (Stanley Price 1977a; Kiszeley 1978; Meiklejohn et al. 1992). At Sotira the practice of artificial cranial deformation was absent from the human remains (only 7 individuals were found) but at Khirokitia out of the approximately 200 human remains, 39% were found with deformed crania (Angel 1961; Domurad 1986). Although the accepted view is the Neolithic culture of Cyprus was relatively uniform, there are still some differences between sites. These differences could signify different groups of settlers from many parts of the mainland.

7.3.1.4. HOUSES AND ARCHITECTURE

The settlement plan from Neolithic Shillourokambos was derived from PPNA in Syria and according to Peltenburg: "...Tenta (Neolithic Cyprus)[1] faithfully repeats a Syrian PPNA hierarchical settlement pattern." (Peltenburg et al. 2001:55). Even though the round houses from later 7th millennium Tenta and Khirokitia are definitely different from the rectilinear houses found on the mainland during the same epoch (Todd 1986). Evidence from dating suggests the round buildings, which were popular in Aceramic Neolithic Cyprus, remained the custom long after rectangular buildings on the mainland replaced them. This could be a sign of the insularity of the Cypriot culture during this time period (7th millennium) (Todd 1986).

Todd believes the culture on Cyprus in the Aceramic Neolithic period (7th millennium) was distinctly different from that of the mainland. The level of complexity that existed on the mainland during the Cypriot Neolothic/Chalcolithic transition was not present in Cyprus and the level of complexity that existed during the Aceramic Neolithic was not present at that time either (Todd 1989). Also, wall paintings found at both Tenta and Khirokitia are similar to the ones identified from Çatal Hüyük (Anatolia) and Mureybet in the Euphrates Valley in north central Syria and at Abu Hureyra (also in the same area in Syria) (Todd 1986; Åström 1989).

---

[1] Author's parenthesis

7.3.2. EVIDENCE OF CYPRIOT ARTEFACTS ON THE MAINLAND

There is little evidence of Cypriot artefacts appearing on the mainland. One such find is a stone vessel of Khirokitia type that was found in the Amuq A period (before 6000 BC) at the site of Amuq in northern Syria (plain of Antioch) (Mellaart 1965; Christou 1989).

7.3.3. SUMMARY

By the time of the Khirokitia culture, contact between the mainland had diminished and it seems that Cyprus was 'culturally isolated' from the mainland. Whether this cultural isolation also reflects biological isolation is uncertain. The culture was uniform on the island throughout the Neolithic and Chalcolithic; it is unknown whether the biological affinities were. The evidence presented above shows Cyprus as an island culture that has adopted customs and technology of an earlier time from the mainland and developing independently from it. This idea of an independently evolving culture seems to have been established from the initial colonists and carried through until the Bronze Age when the island's isolation was ended. Simmons sums up this overall impression of Neolithic Cyprus:

> "The Neolithic in Cyprus shares general similarities conforming to subsistence, settlement, architectural, and mortuary patterns characteristic of early village life throughout the Near East. These, however, occur somewhat later, and show only limited parallels with the mainland. Thus the Cypriot Neolithic presents an interesting contrast in the development and spread of Near Eastern Neolithic cultures." (Simmons 1994:1-2)

There is evidence of some trade with the mainland during the Neolithic but that trade was limited in its scope, type and quantity of goods traded. Until the Middle Bronze Age, Cyprus remained culturally independent from the mainland (Georgiou 1979; Simmons 1994).

Many archaeologists have noted that Cilicia and the Amuq plain are geographically closest to Cyprus and may have been a possible location from which the first Cypriots migrated (Myers 1939; Dikaios 1940; Stanley Price 1977a; Sherratt & Sherratt 1991). Migration rarely works in one direction and the Khirokitia pottery found in Tarsus (Cilicia) may be an indication of this return along the original migration route (Anthony 1990). Cilicia is in Anatolia, but there is evidence to suggest that since the Neolithic it has been a region strongly influenced by northern Syria as well as Anatolia (Alkim 1969; Mellink 1989; 1992).

These connections with the mainland ceased at some point during the late Cypriot Neolithic (or early Chalcolithic), suggested by the lack of archaeological evidence. During the Chalcolithic period, even though sites like Tarsus and Mersin were part of the Anatolian culture, they were still influenced through contacts with Halaf and Ubaid cultures of north Syria and north Mesopotamia (Alkim 1969; Akkermans 1989; Mellink 1989; 1992). That cultural influence did not continue to be transmitted to Cyprus. The discovery of Chalcolithic Cypriot Erimi wares found in Tarsus (Early Bronze II Tarsus) suggests however, a reemerged trade link with the mainland (Buchholz 1969; Mellink 1989; 1991).

Another possibility is there are yet undiscovered settlements in Cyprus which may show continuous contact with the mainland throughout the later Neolithic and that the people from Chalcolithic southwest Cyprus represent a more recent immigrant population with biological contacts, but not cultural ones with the mainland. The suggested evidence from the Early Neolithic on Cyprus is the people may have chosen to split with the culture on the mainland. Therefore the insular nature of Cyprus, which many archaeologists refer to, was a product of the Cypriots themselves.

These arguments are meant to reinforce the archaeological evidence, which already suggests a Syrian origin for the Neolithic Cypriots. Much more dental non-metric data must be collected from other sites in Cyprus, Syria, Anatolia and the Levant to create a broader picture of the biological affinities of people from the Neolithic to the Bronze Age.

7.4. LATE NEOLITHIC SOTIRA AND CHALCOLITHIC ERIMI CULTURES

The evidence for describing the Khirokitia culture and the cultural contacts with the mainland has already been discussed. There is clear evidence of continuous cultural continuity between the early Neolithic culture and the later Chalcolithic. A brief summary of these cultures will be presented below (See Appendix 2 for complete Cypriot chronology).

7.4.1. END OF THE KHIROKITIA CULTURE

By approximately 5000 B.C. the successful Khirokitia culture came to an end. There is no evidence for an influx of people to the island or any new culture from the mainland, or evidence of violence or invasion (Domurad 1986). This is important because the Sotira culture, which was first thought to have come from outside the island, shows strong cultural links with the preceding Khirokitia culture (Held 1992). Any immigrants coming from the mainland would have more cultural connections with the people from Chalcolithic Anatolia or the Halaf culture in northern Syria rather than the Khirokitia people of the early Neolithic (Alkim 1969; Mellink 1992; Schwartz 1992). If there were a merging of indigenous and foreign cultures then there would be some evidence from the cultures on the mainland just mentioned. Evidence will be presented,

explaining that Sotira and Chalcolithic cultures have their roots with the ancient indigenous culture and not immigrants.

7.4.2. SOTIRA CULTURE

There is a connection between the Neolithic Khirokitia and Late Neolithic Sotira cultures with a gap of approximately 500 years. Although the transition from the exclusively lithic and ceramic Sotira culture to the later newly copper-using Erimi culture is nearly seamless (Held 1992). The Sotira culture also has the reputation of being uniform throughout the island (Peltenburg 1978; Peltenburg 1985b; Domurad 1986; Held 1992; Peltenburg 1993; Clarke 2001). Peltenburg compares the Late Neolithic sites of Ayios Epiktitos-Vrysi on the north coast and Sotira-Teppes near the south: "…apart from their contrasting topographical features and pottery ornamentation, their homogenous material culture point to the existence of similarily-organised communities throughout most of the island." (Peltenburg 1993:10).

Unlike the earlier Neolithic there is not much evidence of contact between the Sotira culture and the mainland during the Late Neolithic (Peltenburg 1978; Clarke 2001). One of the problems with understanding change in culture from Khirokitia to Sotira is the lack of sites showing a continuous occupation from the earliest part of the Neolithic (Khirokitia) to the end of the Neolithic (Sotira) (Domurad 1986).

The appearance of ceramics in the Sotira culture has allowed for the observation of regional variation. In prehistoric societies regional variation in ceramics, occurs from outside influences, since there is little evidence for such contact during the Late Neolithic, Clarke suggests this regional variation was the product of:

> "Interaction, based upon kinship and inter-marriage, work-groups, hunting parties etc. would have created intricate social relations that would have been negotiated on both an individual and group level. Competition for resources within site catchment areas may also have contributed to the creation of social and economic boundaries." (Clarke 2001:78)

One can only assume these interactions would have continued into the Chalcolithic. It is possible these interactions are reflected in the Chalcolithic dental affinities, presented above, which may help to explain the local variation between Lemba and Mosphilia.

7.4.3. ERIMI CULTURE

The Erimi culture is based on the site with the same name (Pambolula-Erimi) in the south, near the modern city of Limassol (Bolger 1987; 1988). The Erimi settlements have been found all around the island with many cultural similarities (Peltenburg 1978). There are many similarities between Erimi and other Sotira culture sites such as Sotira-Teppes and Ayios Epiktetos-Vrysi (Peltenburg 1978; Bolger 1988; 1989; Campo 1994). The Sotira culture has been known for regional distinctions, which is repeated with the Erimi culture (Bolger 1988; 1989). With the Erimi culture there was also a shift to the west of the island, which was thought to have been uninhabited during the Neolithic (Maier & Karageorghis 1984; Bolger 1986; Domurad 1986). Recent excavations have found a Neolithic site approximately 20 km east of Paphos and approximately 5 km north by northwest of Souskiou (Simmons 1994). The site called Kholetria Ortos is a large Aceramic Neolithic site and is situated along the Xeropotamos River and relates culturally to the other Aceramic Neolithic sites found in Cyprus (Simmons 1994). This suggests the Khirokitia culture was also present in southwest Cyprus that may be link to the Chalcolithic sites in this study.

The emergence of the Erimi culture is believed to have begun with the appearance of new settlers (perhaps from Tarsus), as evidenced by new styles of figurines, pottery, and the first copper objects (Bolger 1988). The Erimi culture has definite connections with the Neolithic with regards to pottery styles and architectural traditions (Domurad 1986). It is also believed these new people were incorporated into the existing culture. Accepting the idea of immigrants to Cyprus during the Chalcolithic still does not alter the evidence there were very few connections with the mainland (Stanley Price 1980). This idea is also supported by other archaeologists, such as Held (1993) and Swiny (1986:29) who states that during the Chalcolithic Cyprus seems "...to have thrived in almost splendid isolation.". It has also been suggested that an indigenous evolution of culture, religious symbols and technology occurred without influence from outside Cyprus (Peltenburg 1990; Held 1992; 1993; Knapp 1994).

These are two contrary views, one of Cyprus being totally isolated from the mainland during the Chalcolithic and the other being some isolation with people arriving in Cyprus. If Cyprus was colonised as recently as the Chalcolithic then the dental non-metric analysis could support this migration theory with the close biological connection to Syria, presented in this study. Since there are no data older than the Chalcolithic in this study this theory seems possible. The lack of significant cultural contacts with the mainland since the Neolithic makes this recent migration theory more unlikely. To identify any new biological material in the samples in this study, there would have to be enough biological material to make an appreciable difference in the overall biological affinities of the population (Scott & Turner 1997).

The evidence presented in Chapter 2 clearly shows a homogenous culture among the three sites of southwest Chalcolithic Cyprus that seems to fit well with the homogeneous biological nature of the samples. This is also in agreement with the theory of related biology and related culture and according to Ossenberg: "...where cultural, geographical and biological data do concur the evidence for group relationships is considerably reinforced." (Ossenberg 1977:97). Following this, the homogeneity of the Erimi culture extends throughout Cyprus suggesting the biological homogeneity may also existed throughout the island. The question arises, is this close biological similarity representative of all western Cyprus or even the entire island? The premise of this thesis expresses the opinion this should not be automatically assumed, but when there is biological evidence to support this idea then it can be a reasonable assumption. Since there are no other dental non-metric samples that can be tested from other sites in Cyprus during the Chalcolithic, then the cultural remains must be examined.

7.4.4. EVIDENCE FOR CONTACT WITH THE MAINLAND

Red-on-White and Red and Black Streak Burnished Ware have been found at Tarsus in Anatolia, providing evidence of contact with Cyprus not earlier than 2700 B.C. (Swiny 1986; Mellink 1991). During the Chalcolithic, copper artefacts were first identified and even though Cyprus is known for copper, it is possible the early copper found on sites was actually from the mainland (Tylecote 1981; Swiny 1986; Gale 1991). This is more evidence for external contact with Anatolia but it does not explain the degree of contact. The copper mentioned above has been found at the following sites between the years 3500 to 2500B.C.: Erimi, Souskiou, Lemba, Mosphilia and Mylouthkia (Gale 1991). In contrast from the mid-fifth millennium around Anatolia, the Levant and even the Balkans there is much more copper of better grade than found on Cyprus for that later time, therefore even this contact with the mainland was of a limited scale (Gale 1991).

7.4.5. END OF THE CHALCOLITHIC

Nearing the end of the Chalcolithic there is an increase in the overseas contact with the mainland (Dikaios & Stewart 1962; Åström & Åström 1972; Watkins 1981; Swiny 1986; Knapp 1994). The appearance, for the first, of pithos jars at Mosphilia is clear indication of foreign contact on Cyprus during the end of the Chalcolithic onward (Peltenburg et al. 1998). Many archaeologists believe the changes that took place at the end of the Chalcolithic were the result of local initiatives possibly with some external contacts (Watkins 1981; Swiny 1986; Peltenburg 1982; 1985a; 1990; 1991; Knapp 1994).

7.4.6. SUMMARY

After studying the prehistory of Cyprus it is understandable this island would remain biologically as well as culturally isolated but the fact that the mainland sample still shares many similarities suggests there has been little change there. It is unknown when this contact could have ended and the difference from the beginning of the Sotira culture to the time period of the samples from middle and late Chalcolithic Cyprus is less than 2000 years (Appendix 2). This time period is short enough in terms of dental evolution, in which there would be very little change from the parent population. Since dental traits take such a long time to change it might be more appropriate to view the trait frequencies as indicators of ancient contact – therefore it should come as no surprise there is still a connection to the mainland. However, the lack of evidence for significant cultural contact with the mainland since the Neolithic make this theory the most likely given the available evidence. The archaeological evidence supports the theory of an island that is not influenced by the cultural and social changes occurring around it in the Near East. If this truly is the case of a culturally and biologically isolated island before the Bronze Age, then Cyprus presents a unique place to follow the internal change of culture, without much obvious cultural or biological influence from outside.

The biological connection with the mainland as evidenced by the dental non-metrics is unsurprising given the slow rate of change for dental traits. More importantly, since the Neolithic (or later) the sample from Jeralbus which is not in close proximity to Cyprus, still shares many traits which were part of the initial wave of colonisation(s). The surprise is that given the amount of change that should have occurred on the mainland (since it is not geographically isolated), in a few thousand years the mainland population still shows similarities with this ancient colonisation, given the many cultural changes occurring on the mainland since the Neolithic.

7.5. MIDDLE BRONZE GREECE AND LATE BRONZE AGE CYPRUS

The archaeological evidence suggests there was contact between the Aegean and Cyprus from the middle Bronze to the late Bronze Age (LBA). The analyses from the non-metric traits suggest there was a strong relation between the LBA and Chalcolithic sites. Table 6.2 ($D.\theta$) and 6.3 (MMD) show a similar pattern between these five samples, with some differences. The mixed pattern emerging from the samples may be due to small samples or background noise. Or they might be representative of the interaction Cyprus was engaged in between the civilisations of east and west (Gjerstad et al., 1934). This scenario suggests a mixture of cultural and biological influences coming from the east (Canaan and Tarsus) and from the west (Mycenae and Crete), with a core local population also contributing to the gene pool. The amount and intensity of biological influence coming from external sources will vary and is unknown. Also, the sites (in this study) represented in the LBA (Ayios Iakovos and Enkomi) are not representative of 'average' populations (4.5). They are underrepresented in children and they are all from large wealthy rock cut tombs, that held the elite or ruling class, which may be different from the 'average' population. This is in contrast to the samples from Lemba and Mosphilia that are more representative of the 'average' person (4.2). The LBA samples will be more important when they compared with other LBA Cypriot settlements and more generalised ones. The custom of artificial cranial deformation will also be discussed, in the context that it appears in large frequency in Late Bronze Age Cyprus but not in Greece.

7.5.1. DENTAL NON-METRIC EVIDENCE

According to the results from the MMD and $D.\theta$ comparisons, the sites from northeast LBA Cyprus seem to show a mixed relation to Middle Bronze Age Greece. Figure 6.1 ($D.\theta$) shows Enkomi with some similarity to Lerna, while Ayios Iakovos is more dissimilar and Asine is the most dissimilar. Figure 6.1 shows Ayios Iakovos displaying more similarity to Asine and Enkomi while Lerna is the most dissimilar. Northeast Cyprus does not represent a homogenous biological group, although there are cultural similarities. This is clearly different from the pattern in southwest Cyprus. Ayios Iakovos and Enkomi have a mixed pattern of relatedness to each other and to southwest Cyprus. There are some connections between the Chalcolithic and LBA that are not clear at this time. With so few samples it is prudent to proceed with caution to conclude anything definite. The non-metric connections to MBA Greece may also represent a biological influx from the Aegean. It may perhaps be this combination from east and west that is creating a mixed picture among the LBA samples.

While there is a pattern of similarity between the LBA and Chalcolithic sites, their relationship to MBA Greece is more mixed and not as straightforward. It should be pointed out these 2 samples are small and not very reliable, but they may still help to understand their relationship to Chalcolithic Cyprus. One main difference from the Chalcolithic samples is how these two sites do not share many similarities to each other as they do to the Chalcolithic samples. This suggests a difference in the relation between the northeast sites and Greece. Unlike southwest Cyprus that is biologically homogeneous, these sites are quite different but each shows relations to its southwest neighbours and some connection to Jeralbus. There is also biological similarity between southwest Cyprus and the mainland, suggesting no matter how much the sites will differ from each other, they still share some affinities with the ancient parent population.

Although Lerna and Asine are considered part of the same cultural group in MBA Greece, their dental affinities do not represent a homogeneous group. Given that Asine is too small a sample to allow adequate comparison to the much larger Lerna sample, these conclusions should not be considered conclusive.

7.5.2. CONTACTS WITH THE AEGEAN DURING THE EARLY BRONZE AGE

Just as there is little or no direct evidence between Cyprus and the Near East during the Chalcolithic, there is little evidence of Aegean trade or contact with Cyprus until the end of the 3rd and early 2nd millennium B.C. (Renfrew 1972; Mantzourani & Theodorou 1989; Lambrou-Phillipson 1990; Broodbank 2000). From the second millennium onwards there was a maritime network extending from the Aegean to Egypt (Broodbank 2000). By the Late Bronze Age there is an increase in Mycenaean pottery found in the Near East relating to increased trade (Renfrew 1972; Karageorghis 1990; Lambrou-Phillipson 1990; Broodbank 2000).

7.5.3. CONTACTS WITH THE AEGEAN DURING THE LATE BRONZE AGE

From the Middle and Late Bronze Age the Aegean culture begins to expand into the eastern Mediterranean (Åström 1969; Renfrew 1973). During the Late Helladic IIIA and B periods large quantities of Mycenaean pottery, from sites in the Near East, was found and much of it was being produced on Cyprus where the pottery was indistinguishable from that of the Mycenaean homeland (Renfrew 1972; Catling 1991; Sherratt & Sherratt 1991; Sherratt 1992). The quantity of Mycenaean pottery found at Enkomi and other prominent Cypriot settlements suggested to many archaeologists these were indeed colonists who settled in Cyprus making these vast quantities of ceramics (Bartoněnk 1973; Georgiou 1979; Karageorghis 1982; Åström 1991; Catling 1991; Bunimovitz 1998; Iacovou 1998). According to Lambrou-Phillipson:

> "The earliest Mycenaean pottery appears during the LC IB (ca. 1450-1400), when Mycenaean IIB and IIIA1 pottery is present in significant quantities. This material occurs at Hala Sultan Teke, Maroni, Arpera on the south coast, at Enkomi and Milia (Ayios Iakovos) in the east, and Nicosia in the center." (Lambrou-Phillipson 1990:92).

Regarding this supposed migration of Mycenaeans to Cyprus: "…although immigration from the Aegean to Cyprus may well have taken place relatively regularly throughout the Late Cypriot II-IIIA period, such immigration is archaeologically invisible…"(Sherratt 1992:326). If there was such Mycenaean migration to Cyprus, the non-metric evidence from LBA Cyprus might be more similar to the MBA Greece than the current evidence shows.

Laboratory analysis has shown the majority of Mycenaean pottery in Cyprus in Late Cypriot II was imported from the Argolid (Lambrou-Phillipson 1990). However by the later thirteenth century, Cypriot potters were imitating Mycenaean ware (Lambrou-Phillipson 1990; Catling 1991; Sherratt 1994). Along with the Mycenaean influence on the ceramic assemblage during the Late Bronze Age, there is also evidence for a continuation of older Cypriot ceramic traditions that combined with Mycenaean designs (Kling 1989). Except for ceramic wares, all other aspects of Mycenaean culture were absent on Cyprus (before Late Cypriot III), with the exception of Enkomi where a silver bowl and two silver vases have been found (Lambrou-Phillipson 1990). This may also suggest no migration (of significant proportion) occurred. According to Sherratt: "Whatever the origin of the pottery of Mycenaean type found in Cyprus at this time is widely accepted what it is unlikely to have been the product of Aegean colonists on the island." (Sherratt 1994:36). The spread of culture from east to west may have occurred by the copying of one's neighbour and adopting certain aspects of a material culture (Sherratt & Sherratt 1991). This mimicking of culture can include the demand by local populations of certain exotic goods, which in turn become basic necessities in which a population expects and demands. This might explain the already mentioned import of Mycenaean ceramics on Cyprus, and later, the local production of them to sustain this demand (Shearratt 1994).

Along with ceramic styles, Cypriots also adopted Mycenaean tomb types. It has been suggested the Mycenaean style tholos tombs found at Enkomi (15th century B.C.) were of Mycenaean origin, of Greeks who had migrated to Cyprus (Courtois 1969). According to Iacovou, this idea of a Mycenaean cultural presence in some towns on Cyprus has been interpreted as an enculturation of Cypriot society:

> "The tangible result of these changes in Cyprus point towards the Late Mycenaean parentage of the tomb type and the painted ware and disclose the identity of the leading ethnic element in Cyprus at the beginning of the Iron Age. A pan-Cyprian Greek identity was formed in the 11th century." (Iacovou 1998:338).

It should be noted this enculturation is mainly based on pottery assemblages. Just as more Mycenaean artefacts appeared on Cyprus from Late Helladic III onward there is evidence for Cypriot objects on mainland Greece and the Aegean Islands earlier in Late Helladic I (Lambrou-Phillipson 1990). Since there is little evidence of Cypriot artefacts in Greece it has been suggested the Greeks imported perishable goods or raw materials like copper (Catling 1991).

During the period between 1400 – 1200 B.C. Cyprus entered a new phase of urbanisation with important towns emerging along the routes of the copper belt, along the edges of the Troodos Mountains to the sea. Towns such as Enkomi and Kition as well as others along the coast emerged as administrative centres for the distribution of copper (Georgiou 1979; Stanley Price 1980; Sherratt & Sherratt 1991). Was this phase due to immigrating Mycenaeans who arrived in Cyprus with a desire for their own pottery, which they then had imported from Greece in large quantities and began manufacturing it themselves? Or did Cyprus naturally start to change, as a result of expanded foreign contacts, which attracted Mycenaean wares and then immigrants (Åström 1969)? According to the non-metric analysis Enkomi does show some similarity to Lerna while Ayios Iakovos does not. The samples from LBA Cyprus are not representative of a whole settlement (4.6), and may not be representative of all of the people who lived there. Therefore it should be noted these samples are not representative of the biological affinities of the entire site. Until more dental traits are studied from other sites from Middle and late Bronze Cyprus, this question will remain.

7.5.4. CONTACTS WITH THE MAINLAND IN THE LATE BRONZE AGE

There is evidence for strong relations with the Levant, Syria and especially with Carchemish from the Middle and Late Bronze (Åström 1969; Georgiou 1979; Åström 1989; 1991; Fischer 1999). Georgiou states: "The existence of a shrine to a Syrian goddess on Cyprus might imply that there were enough Syrian residents (rather than transients such as merchants or sailors) on Cyprus to support such a building."(Georgiou 1979:93).

Enkomi for example, became more prominent in the expanded trade network with the Near East during Middle Cypriot III (1700-1600/1550) and by Late Cypriot I (1550-1400)(Georgiou 1979). While Mycenaean colonists may have influenced Enkomi, Åström suggests the site of Hala Sultan Tekke may have been biologically influenced from Canaan in the Levant (Åström 1991). There is also evidence of Cypriot pottery dominating the imports from the end of the Middle Bronze to the Late Bronze IIA (and possibly later) at the site of Tell Abu al-Kharaz in Jordan (Fischer 1999).

This evidence for contacts with the east may not only be economic exchange, but may have also resulted in biological exchange. There may have occurred a mixture of biology from the east as well as the west that helped to transform Cyprus in the Late Bronze Age. While there is some similarity between Enkomi and Ayios Iakovos and Jerablus with the $D.\theta$ analysis (Figure 6.2) the MMD analysis (Figure 6.3) is in question because both values are not significant and can not be compared with the results from the first equation. Therefore the evidence from these samples is not clear. Analysing more samples from Cyprus as well as from sites around the Levant and the Near East will help to understand the biological affinities of the people of LBA Cyprus.

7.6. ARTIFICIAL CRANIAL DEFORMATION

Throughout this study the theme of artificial cranial deformations on Cyprus kept appearing in the background research, as well as in some of the samples studied. A short discussion would be helpful to understand its implications relating to the discussion of contact and migration throughout the long history of Cyprus. Artificial cranial deformation is a physiological response to a cultural custom and falls within the range of this study.

Artificial cranial deformation is known from the Neolithic Near East, Levant and eastern Anatolia and has been thoroughly documented elsewhere (Hasluck 1947; Kiszelv 1978; Özbek 2001). It is not known from Mersin and Tarsus, two sites in Anatolia that may have close links to Cyprus from throughout the Neolithic (Domurad 1986; 1989). This custom is not consistent throughout the ancient Near East but it seems to have been prevalent over a large expanse of time.

Artificial cranial deformation is prominent in the human remains from Khirokitia (Neolithic I), but absent from Sotira (Neolithic II). This could be the result of too small a sample from Sotira (Angel 1961; Domurad 1986). It has also been found at the following Chalcolithic sites in eastern Turkey: Değimentepe (second half of the 5th millennium B.C.)(Özbek 2001); Kurban Höyük (Alpagut 1986) and Şeyh Höyük (contemporary with the Tell Halaf culture of northern Mesopotamia and Syria) (Şenyürek & Tunakan 1951).

It was believed that the people from Sotira were an immigrant population who merged with the indigenous population (Angel 1961; Domurad 1989). The appearance of a new group of people who did not practice cranial deformation would explain this discontinuity with the Khirokitia culture. However at that time, the Sotira culture still has more in common with Khirokitia than the mainland cultures in the Near East (Özbek 2001).

Chalcolithic southwest Cyprus has very few observable complete crania, but the effects of cranial deformation in the form of ossicles in the cranial sutures as well as the shapes of the individual parts of the skull are easy to identify and document (Bennett 1965; Ossenberg 1970; Gottlieb 1978). The Stature and Non-metrics Chapter presents the frequency of these traits for all samples in this study. It clearly shows the absence of ossicles in the cranial sutures from southwest Cyprus (Figure 5.1). Although there is evidence from Jerablus of a slight presence of ossicles at the lambda suture (Figure 5.1) there is no evidence of cranial deformation.

It also may be absent from other sites from Middle Bronze Age Cyprus such as Mesoyi-Katarrakis and Marki-Alonia. There are very few human remains from these sites and there is no mention of cranial deformation in the published reports (Herscher and Fox 1993; Moyer 1997). During the

LBA there is a 're-appearance' of the custom at Hala Sultan Tekke, Kition, Ayios Iakovos and Enkomi (Schwartz 1976; Fischer 1986; this volume).

Cranial deformation also does not appear in Middle Bronze Greece (Angel 1971a; Domurad 1989). This absence of cranial deformation from Greece is not in agreement with the theory of Mycenaean settlers on Cyprus during the LBA, where the custom has a high frequency. This custom is socially determined and is not biological and is more informative about a population's social customs rather than their biological affinities. However the point to be made here is how complex migration can be for both migrants and locals, and the way each group deals with biological and cultural continuity.

7.6.1. SUMMARY

Having only a limited sample from the LBA, it is less likely that Cyprus was strongly influenced biologically by 'colonists' from different cultures around the eastern Mediterranean (Åström 1969; Sherratt & Sherratt 1991). Unlike the lack of contacts between Neolithic/Chalcolithic and the Late Bronze Age, Cyprus had contacts from all around the eastern Mediterranean that could have influenced the cultural and biological make up of Cyprus. The non-metric analysis may be showing some of the interaction between the indigenous population of Cyprus and the possible inclusion of biological material from east and west.

CHAPTER 8

CONCLUSION

The principal aim of this study has been accomplished. The biological affinities of the populations in this study have been identified and are available for use by other researchers. This study is important is because it is the first of its kind conducted on the Bronze Age in the eastern Mediterranean. It represents the first picture of the biological affinities through the Bronze Age in 3 different countries. It gives the first evidence on the kinds of biological differences there may be between the different peoples.

Another aim of this study was to examine the biological affinities of these populations in the context of cultural movement in relation to biology. This was within the context of the six questions posed in the Introduction (1.2) using the non-metric and demographic data in this study. With only eight sites the conclusions are tentative. First, in the case of southwest Cyprus, a common culture and common biological affinities are in concordance. This agrees with the statement by Ossenberg: "…where cultural, geographical and biological data do concur the evidence for group relationships is considerably reinforced."(Ossenberg 1977:97). Second, the differences between the site types in southwest Cyprus seem to have had an effect on the demographic distribution and possibly on the dental non-metric results. The exclusion of children and infants from Souskiou identifies a social trend among the people buried there and this clearly will have an effect on the biological affinities. Also, Souskiou being a regional cemetery has affected the distribution of dental non-metric traits to include a much wider catchment area than either Lemba or Mosphilia. Third, the 'rules' governing who is buried at Souskiou and who is excluded, is dictated by age to some degree while there are still other social factors affecting the inclusion of certain people. Fourth, the sites from northeast Cyprus (Ayios Iakovos and Enkomi) do not represent a homogeneous biological group, while being very similar culturally. This is clearly different from the pattern in southwest Cyprus. Fifth, while there is some biological connection between LBA and Chalcolithic Cyprus, it is not consistent between the $D.\theta$ and the MMD and may be due to either too small a sample size (in LBA Cyprus) or actually showing a mixture of new traits coming from Syria and Greece. More samples are definitely needed to help address this question. Lastly, Lerna and Asine are part of the same cultural group in MBA Greece, yet their dental affinities do not represent a homogeneous group. Given that Asine is too small a sample to allow for adequate comparison to the much larger Lerna sample, these conclusions should not be considered conclusive.

Another interesting conclusion from this study is the apparent biological relatedness between southwest Cyprus and Syria. In this case if only an archaeological comparison was made, then there would be no connection between these two groups. The biological relation suggests there might be ancient connections between the mainland still present by the Chalcolithic or even gene flow where there is no culture transmission.

An important point concerning these differences is in each case, there might be a relation between sites that are close geographically and not close biologically. Also, biological affinities have much to do with ancestors and mating practices and should not be considered a means of defining a population. I believe it is culture that defines populations, and it is culture linked with tradition and custom, which may affect biological affinity.

Initially this study sought to determine the biological affinities of various samples to use as the basis for establishing a set of criteria not based on culture to define a group. Assuming a biological group is an extension of a cultural group, which has already been determined, the archaeologist uses mainly cultural remains and assumes a homogeneous population from those cultural artifacts. The assumption of cultural, equating to biological homogeneity is a circular assumption. In this study this assumption is also made but with caution, as the basis for a cultural and biological group. The statement and warning by Cavalli-Sforza & Cavalli-Sforza is something that should be headed when these kinds of studies are done:

> "Our first attempt to establish a link between archaeology and genetics was an out-and-out failure. The results showed clearly that there is no particular resemblance between the Sardinians and the people of Puglia, who are in fact, exactly like the other inhabitants of southern Italy. This failure taught me an important lesson: cultural similarities alone are unreliable indicators of genetic similarities." (Cavalli-Sforza & Cavalli-Sforza 1995:128)

This is a problem archaeologists have faced in the past with their assessment of culturally related groups. In the future when other studies such as this one are carried out, samples should be chosen on the basis of geographical and cultural relations to each other and not from a preconceived idea of what constitutes a probable relation to the study sample. In the case of this study, Syria was included simply as an outlying sample and was not expected to feature so prominently in this study. From what was understood in the differences between the culture and geographical distance of Syria and Chalcolithic Cyprus. There was little expectation for this influential site in the Euphrates River Valley, which is clearly at a different level of civilization, have any biological relation with Chalcolithic Cyprus. The inclusion of Syria in this study challenged my preconceptions and allowed me to consider unlikely possibilities, which is what archaeologists should always be attempting to do.

8.1 RECOMMENDATIONS FOR FUTURE RESEARCH

Although the aim of this study was to focus on Cyprus and its relations to the region, the results of this study have suggested other avenues of research, not only related to Cyprus. From the results of the analysis and the discussion of this study, there are three main recommendations, which I can suggest for further study to better understand the biological and cultural affinities of these sites and of the eastern Mediterranean:

1. To further the understanding of southwestern Cyprus during the transition from the late Chalcolithic to the Early Bronze I recommend three courses of study to be pursued:

   i. An anthropological study of other sites contemporary with other sites around Cyprus to gage the homogeneity of the population.

   ii. An examination of the Early Bronze Age population to see if the new culture had biological influences from Anatolia as the cultural influence would suggest. This study would also benefit from an examination of similar age sites on the mainland in Syria/Levant as well as Anatolia.

   iii. A study of Neolithic samples from Cyprus and the mainland to determine if the biological affinities of the Chalcolithic peoples were present during the first major migration to the island in the 6th millennium. The large skeletal sample at Khirokitia would be an excellent sample to start with.

2. A wider study of the other sites in the Argolid to compare to Lerna and to address the problem why Asine has such a different biological make up than Lerna. Is it the result of the much smaller Asine dental sample (which may be unreliable) or a real difference in population affinities? Some contemporary sample populations from the Cyclades would make an acceptable out-group for such a comparison.

3. A better understanding of the way Jerablus fits in with the various migrations that have affected the population of Cyprus. By examining sites south along the Syrian coast and west along the Anatolian coast to see if indeed Jerablus is part of a large population for the region and also to see what aspect of this population it represents. In other words if its biological affinities represent the 'standard' for the region. The comparative sites could either be contemporary with Jerablus or earlier.

4. Collect DNA data from any of these samples to compare to the dental non-metric results to see if they correlate. Newer methods of extracting DNA have been developed which would make analysis more reliable (Yang et al. 1998).

Any of these studies would be of great importance and relevance not only for understanding Cyprus further but also for the deeper understanding of migration and cultural connections throughout the eastern Mediterranean. Also, these studies would create a deeper understanding of each of these regions in regards to their own questions and problems. This method can be used as a starting point or guide on how the other studies could be accomplished.

8.2 CONCLUSIONS FROM USING THIS KIND OF DATA

This method is useful when studying fragmentary human remains, which do not need to be concerned with contamination. There are many collections of skeletal material that may have been studied before and are kept hidden away in storage. This method can be applied to remains from older excavations that were studied years ago and forgotten. Dental non-metric traits are also very useful in determining biological affinities at the local level, which has been shown with southwest Cyprus. The statement by Alt and Vach supports this idea: "Odontologic traits fulfill the requirements for kinship analysis to a much higher degree than do non-metric traits of the cranium." (Alt & Vach 1998:539). Non-metric studies are useful but there must be caution when conclusions based on these studies are taken as pure genetic indicators (Saunders 1989). I suggest the results of these studies should be considered in conjunction with archaeological data to assist in identifying or defining groups. It is through the inclusion of non-metric data in skeletal reports where anthropology and archaeology can be used together to identify ancient populations (Robb et al. 2001). I would like to end with a statement that I agree with from Scott and Dahlberg:

> "In sum, while the authors are fully aware of their limitations, we believe dental morphological traits can contribute significantly to studies of human population structure and history." (Scott and Dahlberg 1982:287)

REFERENCES

Acsadi, G. and Nemeskeri, J. 1970. *History of human lifespan and mortality.* Budapest, Akademiai.

Akkermans, P.M.M.G. 1989. Halaf mortuary practices: A survey. In: O.M.C. Haex, H.H. Curvers and P.M.M.G. Akkermans (Eds), To the Euphrates and Beyond: Archaeological Studies in Honour of Maurits N. van Loon. AA Balkema, Rotterdam, pp 75-88

Alkim, U.B. 1969. Anatolia I: From the beginnings to the end of the 2nd millennium BC. Barrie and Rockliff: The Crescent Press, London.

Alpagut, B. 1986. The human skeletal remains from Kurban Hoyuk (Urfa Province). *Anatolica*, 13:149-174

Alt, K.W., Pichler, S., Vach, W., Klíma, B., Vlcek, E. and Sedlmeier, J. 1997. Twenty-five throusand-year-old triple burial from Dolní Vestonice: An ice-age family? *American Journal of Physical Anthropology*, 102:123-131

Alt, K.W. and Vach, W. 1998. Kinship studies in skeletal remains- Concepts and examples. In, *Dental Anthropology: Fundamentals, Limits and Prospects*, eds., Alt, K.W., Rosing, F.W. and M. Teshler Nicola. Springer Wein, pp. 537-554.

Anderson, J.E. 1968. The skeletal biology of earlier populations. In (ed) D.R. Brothwell, D.R. *The skeletal biology of earlier populations.* Pergamon Press, Oxford, pp 135-148.

Angel, J.L. 1945. Skeletal Material from Attica. *Hesperia*, 14:279-363

Angel, J.L. 1946. Skeletal change in ancient Greece. *American Journal of Physical Anthropology*, 4:69-97.

Angel, J.L. 1953. Appendix II. The Human Remains from Khirokitia. In, P. Dikaios, Khirokitia. Final report on the excavations of a Neolithic settlement in Cyprus on behalf of the Department of Antiquities 1936-1946. (Monographs of the Department of Antiquities of the Government of Cyprus. No. 1) Oxford pp 416-30.

Angel, J.L. 1959. Appendix: Early Helladic Skulls from Aghios Kosmas. In, GE Mylonas; *Aghios Kosmas: An Early Bronze Age Settlement and Cemetery in Attica.* Princeton, New Jersey, Princeton University Press, pp 169-179

Angel, J.L. 1961. Appendix 1: Neolithic Crania from Sotira. In, P. Dikaios (ed.) Sotira. (University Museum Monographs, No. 23.) Philidelphia, pp 223-229

Angel, J.L. 1968. Appendix: Human Remains at Karataş. *American Journal of Archaeology*, 72:260-263.

Angel, J.L. 1969. The bases of palaeodemography. *American Journal of Physical Anthropology*, 30:427-237.

Angel, J.L. 1970. Excavations at Karataş-Semayük and Elmali, Lycia, 1969:Appendix-Human Skeletal remains at Karataş. *American Journal of Archaeology*, 74:245-259.

Angel, J.L. 1971a. Lerna: Volume II the people. Smithsonian Institute Press.

Angel, J.L. 1971b. Early neolithic skeletons from Çatal Hüyük: Demography and pathology. *Anatolian Studies*, 21:77-98.

Angel, J.L. 1977. Appendix 5: Human Skeletons. In *Keos: Volume 1 Kephala, a late neolithic settlement and cemetery*, ed. J.E. Coleman, pp. 133-156. American School of Classical Studies, Princeton.

Angel, J.L. 1982. Appendix 1: Ancient skeletons from Asine. In: S Dietz (ed.), Asine II, 1: General stratigraphical analysis and architectural remains. Skrifter utg. Av Svenska Institute I Athen, Stockholm, pp 105-138

Anscombe, F.J. 1948. The transformation of Poisson, binomial and negative binomial data. *Biometrika*, 35:246-254.

Anthony, D.W. 1990. Migration in Archaeology: The baby and the bathwater. *American Anthropologist*, 92:895-914

Åström, P. 1966. SIMA:Excavations at Kalopsidha and Ayios Iakovos in Cyprus. Göteborg, Paul Åströms Förlag 2.

Åström, P. 1969. The Economy of Cyprus and its Development in the IInd Millennium. *Archaeologia Viva*, 2(3):73-80

Åström, P. 1989. Early connections between Anatolia and Cyprus. In: K. Emre, B. Hrouda, M. Mellink, and N. Özgüç (eds.), *Anatolia and the Ancient Near*

East: Studeis in honor of Tahsin Özgüç. Ankara: Türk Tarih Kurumu Basivevi, pp. 15-17.

Åström, P. 1991. Canaanite jars from Hala Sultan Tekke. In: N.H. Gale (Ed), Bronze Age Trade in the Mediterranean. Göteborg, Paul Åströms Förlag 90, pp 14-151

Åström, L. and Åström P. 1972. *The Swedish Cyprus Expedition 1927-1931: Vol IV Part 1D*. Berlingska Boktryckeriet, Lund.

Bang, G. and Hasund, A. 1971. Morphologic characteristics of the Alaskan Eskimo dentition. I: Shovel-shaped incisors. *American Journal of Physical Anthropology*, 35:43-48.

Bang, G. and Hasund, A. 1972. Morphologic characteristics of the Alaskan Eskimo dentition. II:Carabelli's Cusp. *American Journal of Physical Anthropology*, 37:35-39.

Bartoněnk A. 1973. The place of the Dorians in the Late Helladic world. In: R.A. Crossland and A. Birchall (Eds.) 1973 Bronze Age Migrations in the Aegean: Archaeological and Linguistic Problems in Greek Prehistory. Gerald Duckworth and Company Ltd. London, pp 305-311.

Bass W.M. 1987. *Human Osteology: A laboratory and field manual*. Special Publication No. 2 of the Missouri Archaeological Society.

Becker, M.J. 1988. An analysis of the human skeletal remains from necropolis at İkiztepe. İkiztepe I. Türk Tarih Kurumu Basimevi, Ankara, pp 261-275.

Bennett, K.A. 1965. The Etiology and Genetics of Wormian Bones. *American Journal of Physical Anthropology*, 23: 255-260.

Berry, A.C. 1975. Factors affecting the incidence of non-metrical skeletal variants. *Journal of Anatomy*, 120(3):519-535.

Berry, A.C. 1976. The Anthropological value of minor variants of the dental crown. *American Journal of Physical Anthropology*, 45:257-268

Berry, A.C. 1978. Anthropological and Familial studies on minor variants of the dental crown. In (eds) PM Butler and KA Joysey, *Development, Function and Evolution of Teeth*. Academic Press, pp 81-98.

Berry, A.C. and R.J. Berry 1967. Epigenetic variation in the human cranium. *Journal of Anatomy*, 101(2):361-379.

Berry, A.C. and R.J. Berry 1972. Origins and Relationship of the Ancient Egyptians. Based on a study of non-metrical variations in the skull. *Journal of Human Evolution*, 1:199-208.

Berry, R.J. 1963. Epigenetic polymorphism in wild populations of Mus Musculus. *Genetical Research*, 4:193-220

Berry, R.J. 1968. The biology of non-metrical variation in mice and men. In (ed) D.R. Brothwell, *The skeletal biology of earlier populations*. Oxford, Pergamon Press, pp. 103-134.

Berry, R.J. 1979. Section I: Genes and skeletons, Ancient and Modern. *Journal of Human Evolution* 8:669-677.

Berry, A.C., Berry, R.J. and Ucko, P.J. 1967. Genetical change in ancient Egypt. *MAN (n.s.)*, 2: 551-568,

Bolger, D.L. 1987. Is There a Western Cyprus? In: David W. Rupp (ed.), *Western Cyprus Connections. An Archaeological Symposium held at Brock University, St. Catharines, Ontario, Canada. March 21-22, 1986*. Göteborg, Paul Åströms Förlag, pp 69-82.

Bolger, D.L. 1988. *Erimi-Pamboula A Chalcolithic Settlement in Cyprus*. BAR International Series, 443

Bolger, D.L. 1989. Regionalism, cultural variation and the culture-area concept in Later Prehistoric Cypriot studies. In: E. Peltenburg (ed.), Early Society in Cyprus. University of Edinburgh Press, Edinburgh. Pp. 142-152

Broodbank, C. 2000. An Island Archaeology of the Early Cyclades. Cambridge University Press

Brown, T.A. and Brown, K.A. 1992. Ancient DNA and the archaeologist. *Antiquity*, 66:140-23

Brown, T.A. and Brown, K.A. 1994. Ancient DNA: Using molecular biology to explore the past (Review Articles). *BioEssays*, 16(10):719-726

Brown, KA., O'Donoghue, K. and Brown, T.A. 1995. DNA in cremated bones from an Early Bronze Age cemetery in Cairn. *International Journal of Osteoarchaeology*, 5:181-187

Buchholz, H.-G. 1973. Grey Trojan ware on Cyprus and Northern Syria. In; RA Crossland and A Birchall (eds.), Bronze Age Migrations in the Aegean: Archaeological and Linguistic Problems in Greek

Prehistory. Gerald Duckworth and Company Ltd. London, pp 197-187

Buikstra, J.E. 1972. Techniques for coping with the age-regressive nature of non-metric traits. *American Journal of Physical Anthropology*, 37(3):431-432

Buikstra, J.E., Frankenberg, S.R. and Konigsberg, L.W. 1990. Skeletal Biological distance studies in American Physical Anthropology: Recent Trends. *American Journal of Physical Anthropology*, 82:1-7

Bunimovitz, S. 1990. Sea Peoples in Cyprus and Israel: A Comparative Study of Immigration Processes. In; Seymour Gitin, Amihai Mazar, and Ephraim Stern (eds.), Mediterranean Peoples in Transition: Thirteenth to Early Tenth Centuries BCE. In Honor of Professor Trude Dothan. Israel Exploration Society, Jerusalem, pp 103-113

Buxton, L.H.D. 1920. Physical anthropology of ancient and modern Greeks. *Nature,* 106(265):183-185.

Campo, A.L. 1994. Anthropomorphic Representations in Prehistoric Cyprus: A Formal and Symbolic Analysis of Figurines, c.3500-1800 B.C.. SIMA Pocketbook. Göteborg, Paul Åströms Förlag, 109.

Carpenter, J.C. 1976. A comparative study of metric and non-metric traits in a series of modern crania. *American Journal of Physical Anthropology*, 45:337-344

Casalotti, R., Simoni, L., Belledi, M. and Barbujani, G. 1999. Y-chromosome polymorphisms and the origins of the European gene pool. *Proceedings of the Royal Society of London B*, 266:1959-1965

Caskey, J.L. 1954. Excavations at Lerna, 1952-1953. *Hesperia,* 23:3-30.

Caskey, J.L. 1955. Excavations at Lerna, 1954. *Hesperia,* 24:25-49.

Caskey, J.L. 1956. Excavations at Lerna, 1955. *Hesperia,* 25:147-173.

Caskey, J.L. 1957. Excavations at Lerna, 1956. *Hesperia,* 26:142-162.

Caskey, J.L. 1958. Excavations at Lerna, 1957. *Hesperia,* 27:125-144.

Caskey, J.L. 1959. Activities at Lerna, 1958-1959. *Hesperia,* 28:202-207.

Caskey, J.L. 1960. The Early Helladic period in the Argolid. *Hesperia,* 29:285-303.

Caskey, J.L. and Blackburn, E.T. 1997. Lerna in the Argolid. American School of Classical Studies at Athens.

Catling, H.W. 1991. Bronze Age Trade in the Mediterranean: a view. In: N.H. Gale (Ed), Bronze Age Trade in the Mediterranean. Göteborg, Paul Åströms Förlag 90, pp 1-14

Cavalli-Sforza, L.L. and Cavalli-Sforza, F. 1995. The Great Human Diasporas: The History of Diversity and Evolution. Addison-Wesley Publishing Co.

Chamberlain, A.T. 1994. *Human Remains*. London: British Museum Press, London.

Chamberlain, A.T. 2000. Problems and Prospects in Palaeodemography. In *Human Osteology in Archaeology and Forensic Science*. Eds. M. Cox and S. Mays. pp. 101-115. London: Greenwich Medical Media

Charles, R.-P. 1962. Le peuplement de Chypre dans l'antiquité. Étude anthropologique. (Étude Chypriotes, 2.) Paris.

Chikhi, L., Destro-Bisol, G., Bertorelle, G., Pascali, V. and Barbujani, G. 1998. Clines of nuclear DNA markers suggest a largely Neolithic ancestry of the European gene pool. *Proceedings of the National Academy of Science USA*, 95:9053-9058

Christou, D. 1989. The Chalcolithic cemetery 1 at Souskiou-Vathyrkakes. In E Peltenburg (ed.):Early Society in Cyprus. University of Edinburgh Press pp. 82-94.

Clarke, J.T. 2001. Style and Society in Ceramic Neolithic Cyprus. *Levant*, 33:65-80

Coale, A.J. and Demeny, P. 1983. *Regional Model Life Tables and Stable Populations*. 2nd edition, Princeton: Princeton University Press.

Coleman, J.E. 1977. In *Keos: Volume 1 Kephala, a late neolithic settlement and cemetery*, ed. J.E. Coleman, pp. 133-156. American School of Classical Studies, Princeton.

Colsen, I.B., Richards, M.B., Bailey, J.F., Sykes, B.C. and Hedges, R.E.M. 1997. DNA analysis of human skeletons excavated from the Terp of Wijnaldum. *Journal of Archaeological Science*, 24:911-917

Conner, M.D. 1990. Population structure and skeletal variation in the Late Woodland of West-Central Illinois. *American Journal of Physical Anthropology*, 82:31-43.

Coppa, A., Cucina, A., Mancinelli, D., Vargiu, R. and Calgano, J.M. 1998. Dental anthropology of Central-Southern Iron Age Italy: The evidence of Metric versus nonmetric traits. *American Journal of Physical Anthropology*, 107:371-386

Corruccini, R.S. 1972. The Biological relationships of some prehistoric and historic Pueblo populations. *American Journal of Physical Anthropology*, 37:373-388.

Corruccini, R.S. 1974. An examination of the meaning of cranial discrete traits for human skeletal biological studies. *American Journal of Physical Anthropology*, 40:425-446.

Courtois, J-C. 1969. Enkomi-Alasia, Glorious Capital of Cyprus. *Archaeologia Viva*, 2(3):93-112

Croft, P. 1985. Area I: The mammalian fauna. In E Peltenburg (ed.) SIMA: Lemba Archaeological Project Volume 1: Excavations at Lemba Lakkous 1976-1983. Göteborg, Paul Åströms Förlag, pp 98-100.

Crossland, R.A. and Birchall, A. (eds.) 1973. Bronze Age Migrations in the Aegean: Archaeological and Linguistic Problems in Greek Prehistory. Gerald Duckworth and Company Ltd. London.

Cucina, A., Lucci, M., Vargiu, R. and Coppa, A. 1999. Dental evidence of biological affinity and environmental conditions in prehistoric Trentino (Italy) samples from the Neolithic to the Early Bronze Age. *International Journal of Osteoarchaeology*, 9:404-416

De Stefano, D.F. 1973. A study of morphological and genetic distance among four Indian villages of Nicaragua. *Journal of Human Evolution*, 2:231-240

De Villiers, H. 1968. The Skull of the South African Negro. A Biometrical and Morphometrical Study. Witwatersrand University Press, Johannesburg.

Derish, P.A. and Sokal, R.R. 1988. A classification of European populations based on gene frequencies and cranial measurements: A map-quadrant approach. *Human Biology*, 60(5):801-824

Dickinson, O.T.P.K. 1995. *The Aegean Bronze Age*. The Cambridge Ancient History. Cambridge University Press

Dikaios, P. 1940. New light on prehistoric Cyprus. *Iraq*, 7:69-83

Dikaios, P. 1953. Khirokitia. Final report in the excavations of a Neolithic settlement in Cyprus on behalf of the Department of Antiquities 1936-1946. (Monographs of the Department of Antiquities of the Government of Cyprus. No. 1) Oxford.

Dikaios, P. 1961. *Sotira*. University Museum Monographs, No. 23, Philidelphia.

Dikaios, P. and Stewart, J.R. 1962. The Swedish Cyprus Expedition 1927-1931: Vol IV Part 1A.

Dittrick, J. and J.M. Suchey 1986. Sex determination of prehistoric central California skeletal remains using discriminant analysis of the femur and humerus. *American Journal of Physical Anthropology*, 70:3-9.

Domurad, M.R. 1986. The Populations of Ancient Cyprus Ph.D. Unpublished Dissertation, University of Cincinnati.

Domurad, M.R. 1989. Whence the first Cypriots? In E Peltenburg (ed.): Early Society in Cyprus. University of Edinburgh Press, pp. 66-70.

Ducos, P. 2000. The Introduction of Animals by man in Cyprus: An alternative to the Noah's ark model. In, M. Mashkour, A.M. Choyke, H. Buitenhuis and F. Poplin (eds.): Archaeozoology of the Near East IV A: Proceedings of the fourth international symposium on the archaeozoology of southwestern Asia and adjacent areas. ARC Publicatie 32 Groningen, The Netherlands, pp 74-82

Dutta, P.C. 1984. Biological Anthropology of Bronze Age Harrapans: New perspectives. In: J.R. Lukacs (ed.), *The People of South Asia: The Biological Anthropology of India, Pakistan, and Nepal*. Plenum Press, New York, pp 59-75

Eller, E. 1999. Population substructure and isolation by distance in three continental regions. *American Journal of Physical Anthropology*, 108:147-159

Evans, J.D. 1973. The archaeological evidence and its interpretation: some suggested approaches to the problems of the Aegean Bronze Age. In: R.A. Crossland and A. Birchall (Eds.) Bronze Age Migrations in the Aegean: Archaeological and

Linguistic Problems in Greek Prehistory. Gerald Duckworth and Company Ltd. London, pp 17-26.

Evison, M.P., Smillie, D.M. and Chamberlain, A.T. 1997. Extraction of single-copy nuclear DNA from forensic specimens with a variety of post-mortem histories. *Journal of Forensic Sciences* 42:1030-1036.

Feldesman, M.R. and Fountain, R.L. 1996. Race specificity and the femur/stature ratio. *American Journal of Physical Anthropology*, 100:207-224

Finnegan, M. 1974. Discrete non-metric variation of the post-cranial skeleton in man (abstract). *American Journal of Physical Anthropology*, 40:135-136.

Finnegan, M. 1978. Non-metric variation of the infracranial skeleton. *Journal of Anatomy*, 125:23-37.

Finnegan, M. and K. Cooprider 1978. Empirical comparison of distance equations using discrete traits. *American Journal of Physical Anthropology*, 49:39-46.

Fischer, P.M. 1986. SIMA: Prehistoric Cypriot Skulls: A medico-anthropological, archaeological and micro-analytical investigation. Göteborg, Paul Åströms Förlag, 75.

Fischer, P.M. 1999. Tell Abu al-Kharaz, Jordon Valley, and Cyprus: a study of Bronze Age interactions. In: KH Niklasson (ed.), SIMA:Cypriote Archaeology in Göteborg: Papers presented at a symposium on Cypriote archaeology held in Göteborg 20 May 1998 (Pocket-book). Göteborg, Paul Åströms Förlag, 157, pp 41-63

Formicola, V. and Franceschi, M. 1996. Regression equations for estimating stature from long bones of early Holocene European samples. *American Journal of Physical Anthropology*, 100:83-88

Forsén, J. 1992. SIMA: The Twilight of the Early Helladics. A study of the disturbances in east-central and southern Greece towards the end of the Early Bronze Age. Göteborg, Paul Åströms Förlag, Pocket-book 116.

Fountoulakis, M. 1985. The anthropological material of early Helladic cemetery of Manika - Chalkis. Athens.

Francalacci, P, Bertranpetit, J, Calafell, F, Underhill, PA 1996. Sequence diversity of the control region of mitochondrial DNA in Tuscany and its implications for the peopling of Europe. *American Journal of Physical Anthropology*, 100:443-460

Frödin, O. and Persson, A.W. 1938. Asine: Results of the Swedish Excavations 1922-1930

Fürst, C.M. 1930. Zur Anthropologie der Prähistorichen Griechen in Argolis, nebst Beschreibungen einiger älteren Schädel aus historischen Zeit (Lunds Univesitets Årsskrift, N.F., Avd. 2, Bd 26:8 = Kungl. Fysiografiska sällskapets handlingar, N.F., Bd. 41:8), Lund and Leipzig

Fürst, C.M. 1933. Zur Kenntnis der anthropologie der prähistorichen Bevölkerung der Insel Cypern. Lunds Universitets Årsskrift, N.F., Avd. 2, Bd 29, Nr. 6, Lund

Gage, T.B. 2000. Demography. In Sara Stinson, Barry Bogin, Rebecca Huss-Ashmore and Dennis O'Rourke (eds), *Human Biology an Evolutionary and biocultural perspective*. Wiley-Liss, New York, pp. 507-551.

Gale, N.H. 1991. Metals and Metallurgy in the Chalcolithic period. *Bulletin of the American School of Oriental Research*, 282/283:37-61

Garn, S.M. 1966. The evolutionary and genetic control of variability in man. *Ann. N.Y. Acad. Sci.*, 134:602-615

Gejvall, Nils-Gustaf 1977. Appendix II: The human remains in Tomb 13 (and 14). In P. Åstöm (ed.): SIMA: The Curass tomb and other finds at Dendra: Part I: the Chamber Tombs. Göteborg, Paul Åströms Förlag, 4:136-144.

Georgiou, H. 1979. Relations between Cyprus and the Near East in the Middle and Late Bronze Age. *Levant*, 11:84-100.

Gilbert, B.M. and McKern, T.W. 1973. A method for aging the female Os publis. *American Journal of Physical Anthropology*, 38:31-38.

Gilmour, G. 1995. Aegean influences in Late Bronze Age funerary practices in the Southern Levant. In: S. Campbell and A. Green (Eds.), *The Archaeology of Death in the Near East*. Oxbow Monograph 51, Oxbow Books Oxford, pp 155-170.

Gjerstad, E., Lindros, J., Sjöqvist, E. and Westholm, A. 1934. The Swedish Cyprus Expedition 1927-1931: Vol 1.

González, A.M., Brehm, A., Pérez, J.A., Maca-Meyer, N., Flores, A. and Cabera, V.M. 2003. Mitochondrial DNA Affinities at the Atlantic fringe of Europe. *American Journal of Physical Anthropology*, 120:391-404

Gottlieb, K. 1978. Artificial cranial deformation and the increased complexity of the lambdoid suture. *American Journal of Physical Anthropology*, 48:213-214

Green, R.F., J.M. Suchey and D.V. Gokhale 1979. The statistical treatment of correlated bilateral traits in the analysis of cranial material. *American Journal of Physical Anthropology*, 50:629-634

Grewal, M.S. 1962. The rate of genetic divergence of sublines in the C57BL strain of mice. *Genetical Research*, 3:226-237

Grünberg, H. 1952. Genetical studies on the skeleton of the mouse. IV: Quasi-Continuous variations. *Journal of Genetics*, 51(1):95-114.

Guatelli-Steinberg, D., Irish, J.D. and Lukacs, J.R. 2001. Canary islands-north African population affinities: measure of divrgence based on dental morphology. *Homo*, 52(2):173-188.

Hadjisavvas, S. 1977. The archaeological survey of Paphos. A preliminary report. *Report of the Department of Antiquities Cyprus*, pp 222-231

Hanihara, T. 1992. Dental and cranial affinities among populations of East Asia and the Pacific: the basic populations in East Asia, IV. *American Journal of Physical Anthropology*, 88:163-182.

Hasluck, M. 1947. Head-deformation in the near east. *MAN*, 47:130-131.

Haydenblit, R. 1996. Dental variation among four prehispanic Mexican populations. *American Journal of Physical Anthropology*, 100:228-246

Held, S.O. 1992. Colonization and Extinction on Early Prehistoric Cyprus. In: Paul Åström (ed.), Acta Cypria: Acts of the International Congress on Cypriote Archaeology held in Göteborg on 22-24 August 1991 Part 2. Göteborg, Paul Åströms Förlag 2, pp 104-164.

Held, S.O. 1993. Insularity as a modifier of culture change: The case of prehistoric Cyprus. *Bulletin of the American School of Oriental Research*, 292:25-33

Hemphill, B.E., Lukacs, J.R. and Kennedy, K.A.R. 1991. Biological adaptations and affinities of Bronze Age Harappans. In (ed) R.H. Meadow, Harappa Excavations 1986-1990: A Multidisciplinary Approach to third Millennium Urbanism. Prehistory Press, Madison Wisconsin, No. 3 pp. 137-182

Hernández, M, García-Moro, C and Lalueza-Fox, C 1998. Stature estimation in extinct Aónikenk and the myth of Patagonian gigantism. *American Journal of Physical Anthropology*, 105(4):545-551

Herscher, E. and Fox, S.C. 1993. A middle Bronze Age tomb from western Cyprus. *Report of the Department of Antiquities Cyprus*, 69-80

Hershkovitz, I, Latimer, B, Dutour, O, Jellema, LM, Wish-Baratz, S, Rothschild, C and Rothschild, BM 1997. Why do we fail in aging the skull from the sagittal suture? *American Journal of Physical Anthropology*, 103:393-399

Hiernaux, J. 1963. Heredity and Environment: Their influence on Human morphology. A comparison on two independent lines of study. *American Journal of Physical Anthropology*, 21:575-590

Hillson, S.W. 1993. Teeth. Cambridge Manuals in Archaeology. Cambridge University Press

Hillson, S.W. 1996. Dental Anthropology. Cambridge University Press

Hjortsjö, C.-H. 1947. To the knowledge of the prehistoric craniology of Cyprus. (Kungl. Hum. Vetenskapssamfundets I Lund årsberättelse 1946-1947.) Lund.

Hoffman, J.M. 1979. Age estimation from dyaphyseal lengths: two months to twelve years. *Journal of Forensic Sciences*, 24:461-469.

Hoppa, R.D. 1992. Evaluating human skeletal growth: an Anglo-Saxon example. *International Journal of Osteoarchaeology*, 2:275-288

Howell, R.J. 1973. The origins of the Middle Helladic culture. In: RA Crossland and A Birchall (Eds.) *Bronze Age Migrations in the Aegean: Archaeological and Linguistic Problems in Greek Prehistory*. Gerald Duckworth and Company Ltd. London, pp 73-106

Iacovou, M. 1998. Philistia and Cyprus in the Eleventh Century: From a similar prehistory to a diverse protohistory. In; Seymour Gitin, Amihai Mazar, and Ephraim Stern (eds.), Mediterranean Peoples in Transition: Thirteenth to Early Tenth Centuries BCE. In Honor of Professor Trude Dothan. Israel Exploration Society, Jerusalem, pp 332-344

Irish, J.D. 1995. High frequency archaic dental traits in modern sub-Saharan African populations (abstract). *American Journal of Physical Anthropology(Supl)*, 20(182):117.

Irish, J.D. 1997. Characteristic high and low frequency dental traits in Sub-Saharan African populations. *American Journal of Physical Anthropology*, 102(4):455-467.

Irish, J.D. 1998. Ancestral dental traits in recent Sub-Saharan Africans and the origin of modern humans. *Journal of Human Evolution*, 34(1):81-98.

Irish, J.D. 2000. The Iberomaurusian enigma: North African progenitor or dead end? *Journal of Human Evolution*, 39:393-410.

Irish, J.D. and C.G. Turner II 1990. West African dental affinity of Late Pleistocene Nubians: Peopling of the Eurafrican-South Asian triangle II. *Homo*, 41:42-53.

Işcan, M.Y., S.R. Loth and R.K. Wright 1984a. Age estimation from the ribs by phase analysis: White males. *Journal of Forensic Sciences*, 29:1094-1104.

Işcan, M.Y., S.R. Loth and R.K. Wright 1984b. Metamorphosis at the sternal rib end: A new method to estimate age at death in white males. *American Journal of Physical Anthropology*, 65:147-156.

Işcan, M.Y., S.R. Loth and R.K. Wright 1985. Age estimation from the ribs by phase analysis: White females. *Journal of Forensic Sciences*, 30:853-863.

Johnson, A.L. and N.C. Lovell 1994. Biological differentiation at Predynastic Naqada, Egypt: An analysis of dental morphological traits. *American Journal of Physical Anthropology*, 93:427-433.

Karageorghis, V. 1990. The End of the Late Bronze Age in Cyprus. The Pierides Foundation, Imprinta Ltd, Nicosia.

Katz, D. and J.M. Suchey 1986. Age determination of the male Os publis. *American Journal of Physical Anthropology*, 69:427-435

Keen, J.A. 1950. A study of the differences between male and female skulls. *American Journal of Physical Anthropology*, 8:65-79.

Kiszely, I. 1978. The Origins of Artificial Cranial Deformation in Eurasia form the Sixth Millennium B.C. to the Seventh Century A.D. BAR International Series Supplementary 50.

Kling, B. 1989. Local Cypriot features in the ceramics of the Late Cypriot IIIA period. In, E Peltenburg (ed.): Early Society in Cyprus. University of Edinburgh Press, pp. 160-170.

Knapp, A.B. 1994. Emergence, development and decline on Bronze Age Cyprus. In: Clay Mathers and Simon Stoddart (eds.), *Development and Decline in the Mediterranean Bronze Age*. Sheffield Archaeological Monographs 8, JR Collis Publications pp 271-304

Konigsberg, L.W. 2000. Quantitative Variation and Genetics. In: Sara Stinson, Barry Bogin, Rebecca Huss-Ashmore and Dennis O'Rourke (eds), *Human Biology an Evolutionary and biocultural perspective*. Wiley-Liss, New York,pp 135-162

Konigsberg, L.W. and Frankenberg, S.R. 1992. Estimation of age structure in anthropological demography. *American Journal of Physical Anthropology*, 89:235-256

Kósa, F. 1989. Age Estimation from the fetal skeleton. In MY Iscan (ed.): *Age Markers in the Human Skeleton*. Charles C Thomas Publisher, Springfield pp. 21-54.

Krogman, W.M. and M.Y. Işcan 1986. *The Human Skeleton in Forensic Medicine*. Charles C. Thomas Publisher, Springfield, Illinois.

Kurth, G. 1958. Zur stellung der neolitischen menschrest von Khirokitia auf Cypern. *Homo*, 9:20-31

Kurth, G. 1980. Beiträge zur anthropologie und populationbiologie des Nahen Osten aus der Zeit von Mesolithikum bis zum Chalkolithikum. Ein examplarischer Versuch anhand der Serien vom Tell es Sultan in Jericho, Khirokitia/Cypern, Byblos/Libanon, Eridu/Irak und Sialk/Iran. *Bonner Hefte zur Vorgeschitchte*, 21:31-203. Bonn.

Lambrou-Phillipson, C. 1990. SIMA: Hellenorientalia: The Near Eastern presence in the Bronze Age Aegean ca. 3000-1100 B.C. Göteborg, Paul Åströms Förlag, Pocket book 95.

Le Mort, F. 2000. The Neolithic Subadult Skeletons form Khitokitia (Cyprus): Taphonomy and Infant Mortality. *Anthropologie*, 38(1)63-70

Lee, G.T.R and Goose, D.H. 1972. The inheritance of dental traits in a Chinese population in the United Kingdon. *Journal of Medical Genetics*, 9:336-339.

Lovejoy, C.O. 1985. Dental wear in Libben popultion: it's functional pattern and role in the determination of adult skeletal age at death. *American Journal of Physical Anthropology*, 68:47-56.

Lukacs, J.R. and Walimbe, S.R. 1984. Deciduous dental morphology and the biological affinities of a late Chalcolithic skeletal series from Western India. *American Journal of Physical Anthropology*, 65:23-30

Lukacs, J.R. and Hemphill, B.E. 1991. The dental anthropology of prehistoric Baluchistan: A morphometric approach to the peopling of South Asia. In: M.A. Kelly and C.S. Larsen (Eds.), Advances in Dental Anthropology. Wiley-Liss Publications Inc, New York. Pp 77-119.

Lunt, D.A. 1985. Discussion of the human dentitions. In E. Peltenburg (ed.) SIMA: Lemba Archaeological Project Volume 1: Excavations at Lemba Lakkous 1976-1983. Göteborg, Paul Åströms Förlag, 245-249.

Lunt, D.A. 1994. Appendix: Report on human dentitions from Souskiou-Vathyrkakas 1972. In: FG Maier and M-L von Wartburg. Excavations at Kouklia (Palaipaphos). Seventeenth preliminary report: Seasons 1991 and 1992. *Report of the Department of Antiquities Cyprus*, pp 120-129.

Lunt, D.A. 1995. Lemba-Lakkous and Kissonerga-Mosphilia: Evidence from the dentition in Chalcolithi Cyprus. In S Campbell and and A Green (eds.):The Archaeology of Death in the Near East, 56-61.

Lunt, D.A., Peltenburg, E.J. and Watt, M.E. 1998. Chapter 4: Mortuary practices. In; E.J. Peltenburg (ed.), SIMA: Lemba Archaeological Project Volume II.1A: Excavations at Kissonerga-Mosphilia, 1979-1992. Göteborg, Paul Åströms Förlag, pp 65-92.

Maier, F.G. 1973. Excavations at Kouklia (Palaepaphos). Sixth preliminary report; seasons 1971 and 1972. *Report of the Department of Antiquities Cyprus*, pp 186-198

Maier, F.G. and Karageroghis, V. 1984. Paphos. History and Archaeology. Nicosia

Maier, F.G. and Wartburg, M-L. von 1994. Excavations at Kouklia (Palaipaphos). Seventeenth preliminary report: Seasons 1991 and 1992. *Report of the Department of Antiquities Cyprus*, pp 115-119.

Mantzourani, E.K. and Theodorou, A.J. 1989. An attempt to Delineate the sea - routes between Crete and Cyprus during the Bronze Age. In, Vassos Karageorghis (ed.): The Civilizations of the Aegean and their diffusion in Cyprus and the Eastern Mediterranean, 2000-600 B.C: proceedings of an international symposium, 18-24 September, 1989. Pierides Foundation, Larnaca, pp 39-55

Meiklejohn, C., Agelarakis, A., Akkermans, P.A., Smith, P.E.L. and Solecki, R. 1992. Artificial cranial deformation in the Proto-neolithic Near East and its possible origin: evidence from four sites. *Paléorient*, 18(2):83-97

Meindl, R.S. and C.O. Lovejoy 1985. Ectocranial suture closure: A revised method for the determination of skeletal age at death based on the lateral-anterior sutures. *American Journal of Physical Anthropology,* 68:57-66.

Mellaart, J. 1965. Earliest Civilizations of the Near East. Thames and Hudson London.

Mellink, M.J. 1989. Anatolia and foreign relations of the Tarsus in the Early Bronze Age. In: K. Emre, B. Hrouda, M. Mellink, and N. Özgüç (eds.), *Anatolia and the Ancient Near East: Studeis in honor of Tahsin Özgüç*. Ankara: Türk Tarih Kurumu Basivevi, pp 319-331

Mellink, M.J. 1991. Anatolian contacts with Chalcolithic Cyprus. *Bulletin of the American School of Oriental Research*, 282/283:167-175

Mellink, M.J. 1992. Anatolian Chronology. In: R.W. Ehrich (ed.), Chronologies in Old World Archaeology Vol 1. The University of Chicago Press, Chicago and London, pp 207-220

Miles, A.E.W. 1963. Dentition in the estimation of age. *Journal of Dental Research*, 42:255-263.

Milner, G.R., Humpf, D.A. and Harpending, H.C. 1989. Pattern matching of age-at-death distributions in paleodemographic analysis. *American Journal of Physical Anthropology*, 80:49-58

Mitford, T.B. and Iliffe, J.H. 1951. Excavations in Kouklia (old Paphos), Cyprus, 1950. *The Antiquaries Journal*, 31:51-66

Molto, J.E. 1979. The assessment and meaning of intraobserver error in population studies based on discontinuous cranial traits. *American Journal of Physical Anthropology*, 51:333-344.

Moorrees, C.F.A., E.A. Fanning and E.E. Hunt 1963a. Formation and resorption of three deciduous teeth in children. *American Journal of Physical Anthropology*, 21:205-213.

Moorrees, C.F.A., E.A. Fanning and E.E. Hunt 1963b. Age variation of formation stages for ten permanent teeth. *Journal of Dental Research*, 42:1490-1502.

Morant, G.M. 1935. A study of Predynastic Egyptian skulls from Badari based on measurements taken by Miss B.N. Stoessiger and Professor D.E. Derry. *Biometrika* 27:293-309.

Moyer, J. 1997. Human remains from Marki-Alonia, Cyprus. *Report of the Department of Antiquities Cyprus*, pp 111-118.

Myers, J.L. 1939. Recent archaeological discoveries in Asia Minor. *IRAQ*, 6:71-90

Mylonas, G.E. 1934. Excavations at Haghios Kosmas. *American Journal of Archaeology*, 38:258-279.

Mylonas, G.E. 1959. *Aghios Kosmas: An Early Bronze Age Settlement and Cemetery in Attica*. Princeton, New Jersey, Princeton University Press.

Nichol, C.R. 1989. Complex segregation analysis of dental morphological variants. *American Journal of Physical Anthropology*, 78(1):37-59.

Nielsen, O.V. 1970. Human Remains Metrical and non-metrical anatomical variations: The Scandinavian Joint Expedition to Sudanese Nubia. Scandinavian University Books Vol 9.

Nielsen, O.V. 1973. Population movements and changes in ancient Nubia with special reference to the relationship between C-group, New Kingdom and Kerma. *Journal of Human Evolution*, 2:31-46

Niklasson, K.H. 1985. Area I: The Graves and Area II: The Graves. In, E.J. Peltenburg (ed.); SIMA: Lemba Archaeological Project Volume 1: Excavations at Lemba Lakkous, 1976-1983. Göteborg, Paul Åströms Förlag 70:1, pp 43-53 and pp 134-149.

Niklasson, K.H. 1991. SIMA: Early Prehistoric Burials in Cyprus. Göteborg, Paul Åströms Förlag 106

Niklasson, K.H. 1999. LC III pit and shaft graves: explaning the "phenomenon"? (Abstract). In: K.H. Niklasson (ed.), SIMA:Cypriote Archaeology in Göteborg: Papers presented at a symposium on Cypriote archaeology held in Göteborg 20 May 1998 (Pocket-book). Göteborg, Paul Åströms Förlag, 157, pp 97-98

Nissen, H.J. 1988. The Early History of the Ancient Near East 9000-2000 BC. The University of Chicago Press, Chicago and London.

Nordquist, G.C. 1987. Asine in the Argolid: A Middle Helladic Village. Uppsala Studies in Ancient Mediterranean and Near Eastern Civilizations 16. Acta Universitatis Upsaliensis Boreas, Uppsala.

Nordquist, G.C. and Hägg, R. 1996. The History of the Asine Excavations and Collections. 1646 Upps. Univ. GustavianumBok Asine III 1:a spaltkorr, Uppsala

Ossenburg, N.S. 1970. The influence of artificial cranial deformation on discontinuous morphological traits. *American Journal of Physical Anthropology*, 33:357-372.

Ossenberg, N.S. 1976. Within and between race distance in population studies based on discrete traits of the human skull. *American Journal of Physical Anthropology*, 45:701-716.

Ossenberg, N.S. 1977. Congruence of Distance Matricies based on cranial discrete traits, cranial measurements and linguistic-geographic criteria in five Alaskan populations. *American Journal of Physical Anthropology*, 47:93-98

Ossenberg, N.S. 1981. An argument for the use of total side frequencies of bilateral nonmetric skeletal traits in population distance analysis: The regression of symmetry on incidence. *American Journal of Physical Anthropology*, 54:471-479

Özbek, M. 2001. Cranial deformation in a subadult sample from Değirmentepe (Chalcolithic Turkey). *American Journal of Physical Anthropology*, 115:238-244

Peltenburg, E.J. 1978. The Sotira culture: Regional diversity and cultural unity in Late Neolithic Cyprus. *Levant*, 10:55-74

Peltenburg, E.J. 1979. The prehistory of west Cyprus: Ktima lowlands investigation. *Report of the Department of Antiquities Cyprus*, 69-99

Peltenburg, E.J. 1982. Recent Developments in Cyprus. SIMA. Göteborg, Paul Åströms Förlag 16

Peltenburg, E.J. 1985a. SIMA: Lemba Archaeological Project Volume 1: Excavations at Lemba Lakkous, 1976-1983. Göteborg, Paul Åströms Förlag.

Peltenburg, E.J. 1985b. Settlement Aspects of the Later Prehistory of Cyprus: Ayios Epiktitos-Vrysi and Lemba. In, Vassos Karageorghis (ed.), Archaeology in Cyprus. 1960-1985. A.G. Leventis Foundation, Zavallis Press Ltd, Nicosia, pp 92-114

Peltenburg, E.J. 1990. Chalcolithic Cyprus. Cyprus Before the Bronze Age: Art of the Chalcolithic Period. The J. Paul Getty Museum, Malibu, California, pp 5-24.

Peltenburg, E.J. 1991. Local exchange in prehistoric Cyprus: An initial assessment of Picrolite. *Bulletin of the American School of Oriental Research*, 282/283:107-126

Peltenburg, E.J. 1993. Settlement Discontinuity and Resistance to Complexity in Cyprus. *Bulletin of the American School of Oriental Research*, 292:9-23

Peltenburg, E.J. Campbell, S., Croft, P., Lunt, D., Murray, M.A. and Watts, M.E. 1995. Jerablus-Tahtani, Syria, 1992-4: Preliminary Report. *Levant* 27:1-28.

Peltenburg, E.J., Bolger, D., Campbell, S., Murray, M.A. and Tipping, R. 1996. Jerablus-Tahtani, Syria, 1995: Preliminary Report. *Levant*, 28:1-25.

Peltenburg EJ, Campbell S, Carter S, Stephen FMK and Tipping R 1997. Jerablus-Tahtani, Syria, 1996: Preliminary Report. *Levant*, 29:1-18.

Peltenburg, E.J. 1998. SIMA: Lemba Archaeological Project Volume II.1A: Excavations at Kissonerga-Mosphilia, 1979-1992. Göteborg, Paul Åströms Förlag.

Peltenburg, E.J., Colledge, S., Croft, P., Jackson, A., McCartney, C. and Murry, M.A. 2000a. Agro-pastoralist colonists colonization of Cyprus in the 10th millennium BP: initial assessments. *Antiquity*, 74(286):844-853

Peltenburg, E.J., Eastaugh, E., Hewson, M., Jackson, A., McCarthy, A. and Rymer, T. 2000b. Jerablus Tahtani, Syria, 1998-1999: Preliminary Report. *Levant*, 32:53-75

Peltenburg, E.J., Colledge, S., Croft, P., Jackson, A., McCartney, C. and Murry, M.A. 2001. Neolithic dispersals from the Levantine Corridor: a Mediterranean perspective. *Levant*, 33:35-64

Phenice, T.W. 1969. A newly developed visual method of sexing the os pubis. *American Journal of Physical Anthropology*, 30:297-302.

Reese, D. 1996. Cypriot hippo hunters no myth. *Journal of Mediterranean Archaeology*, 9(1):107-112

Relethford, J.H. 1994. Craniometric variation among modern human populations. *American Journal of Physical Anthropology*, 95:53-62

Renfrew, C. 1972. The Emergence of Civilisation The Cyclades and the Aegean in the third millennium B.C. Methuen and Co, London

Renfrew, C. 1973. Problems in the general correlation of archaeological and linguistic strata in prehistoric Greece: the model of autochthonous origin. In: R.A. Crossland and A. Birchall (Eds.), Bronze Age Migrations in the Aegean: Archaeological and Linguistic Problems in Greek Prehistory. Gerald Duckworth and Company Ltd. London, pp 263-279

Reynolds, J., Weir, B.S. and Cockerham, C.C. 1983. Estimation of the coancestry coefficient: Basis for a short-term genetics distance. *Genetics*, 105:767-779

Rightmire, G.P. 1972. Cranial Measurements and Discrete Traits Compared in Distance Studies of African Negro Skulls. *Human Biology*, 44(3):263-276.

Richards, M., Smalley, K., Sykes and Hedges, R. 1993. Archaeology and genetics: Analysing DNA from skeletal remains. *World Archaeology*, 25(1):18-28

Richards, M., Corte-Real, H., Forester, P., Macaulay, V., Wilkinson-Herbots, H., Demaine, A., Papiha, S., Hedges, R., Bandelt, H. and Sykes, B. 1996. Palaeolithic and Neolithic lineages in the European Mitochondrial gene pool. *American Journal of Human Genetics*, 59:185-203

Risdon, D.L. 1939. A study of the cranial and other human remains from Palestine excavated at Tell Duweir (Lachish). *Biometrika*, 31(7):99-166.

Robb, J., Bigazzi, R., Lazzarini, L., Scarsini, C. and Sonego, F. 2001. Social "Status" and Biological "Status": A comparison of Grave goods and skeletal indicators from Pontecagnano. *American Journal of Physical Anthropology*, 115:213-222

Roler, K.L. 1992. Near Eastern dental variation past and present (Unpublished Masters for the Arizona State University)

Rothhammer, F. and Silva, C. 1990. Craniometrical variation among South American prehistoric populations: Climatic, altitudinal, chronological and geographic contributions. *American Journal of Physical Anthropology*, 82:9-17

Rutter, J. 1993. Review of Aegean Prehistory 2: The prepalatial Bronze Age of the Southern and central Greek mainland. *American Journal of Archaeology*, 97:745-797

Safizadeh, M.H. and McKenna, D.R. 1996. Application of multidimensional scaling techniques to facilities layout. *European Journal of Operational Research*, 92:54-62

Saunders, S.R. 1978. *The Development and distribution of discontinuous morphological variation of the human infracranial skeleton.* National Museum of Man mercury Series: Ottawa.

Saunders, S.R. 1989. Non-metric skeletal variation. In M.Y. Iscan and K.A.R. Kennedy (eds.): Reconstructions of life from the skeleton. Alan R. Liss Inc. pp. 95-108.

Saunders, S. and F. Popovich 1978. A family study of two skeletal variants: Atlas bridging and clinoid bridging. *American Journal of Physical Anthropology*, 49:193-204.

Scheur, J.L., J.H. Musgrave and S.P. Evans 1980. The estimation of late fetal and perinatal age from limb bone length by linear and logarithmic regression. *Annals of Human Biology*, 7:257-265.

Schliwa, R., Gilbert, K., Walter, H. and Dannewitz, A. 1983. Serological-genetic investigations on some populations of the Northern Aegean Sea (Greece). *Journal of Human Evolution*, 12:769-733

Schulte-Campbell, C.C. 1986. Human Remains. In: I.A. Todd (ed.) SIMA: Vasilikos Valley Project 1: The Bronze Age cemetery in Kalavasos village. Göteborg, Paul Åströms Förlag 71(1):168-179.

Schwartz, G.M. 1992. Syria, ca. 10,000-2000 B.C. In: R.W. Ehrich, (ed.), Chronologies in Old World Archaeology Vol 1. The University of Chicago Press, Chicago and London, pp 221-243

Schwartz, J.H. 1976. Appendix I: Skeletal Remains. In P Åström, DM Bailey and V Karageorghis (eds.):SIMA: Hala Sultan Tekke: Excavations 1897-1971. Göteborg, Paul Åströms Förlag 45(1):90-92

Schwartz, J.H. 1995. *Skeleton Keys.* Oxford University Press.

Sciulli, P.W. 1990. Cranial metric and discrete trait variation and biological differentiation in the terminal Late Archaic of Ohio: The Duff site cemetery. *American Journal of Physical Anthropology*, 82:19-29.

Scott, G.R. and Dahlberg, A. 1982. Microdifferentiation in tooth crown morphology among Indians of the American southwest. In: B. Kurtén (ed.), Teeth: Form, Function, and Evolution. Columbia University Press, New York. Pp. 259-291

Scott, G.R. and Alexandersen, V. 1992. Dental morphological variation among Medieval Greenlanders, Icelanders, and Norwegians. In: P. Smith and E. Techernov (Eds.), Structure, Function and Evolution of Teeth. Freund Publishing House Ltd, London. Pp. 467-490

Scott, G.R. and C.G. Turner II 1997. *The Anthropology of modern human teeth: Dental morphology and its variation in recent human populations.* Cambridge University Press.

Şenyürek, M.S. 1947. A note on the duration of life of the ancient inhabitants of Anatolia. *American Journal of Physical Anthropology*, 5(1):55-66.

Şenyürek, M.S. 1955. A note on the long bones of Chalcholithic age from Şeyh Höyük. *Türk Tarih Kurumu Belleten*, 19:247-270.

Şenyürek, M.S. and S. Tunakan 1951. The skeletons from Şeyh Höyük. *Türk Tarih Kurumu Belleten*, 15:439-445.

Shennan, S. 1997. *Quantifying Archaeology.* University of Iowa Press, Iowa City (Second Edition)

Sherratt, E.S. 1992. Immigration and Archaeology: Some Indirect Reflections. In: P Åström (ed.), Acta Cypria: Acts of the International Congress on Cypriote Archaeology held in Göteborg on 22-24 August 1991 Part 2. Paul Åströms Förlag pp. 316-347

Sherratt, E.S. 1994. Patterns of Contact between the Aegean and Cyprus in the 13th and 12th centuries B.C. *Archaeologia Cypria*, 3:35-43

Sherratt, A. and Sherratt, S. 1991. From luxuries to commodities: the nature of Mediterranean Bronze Age trading systems. In: N.H. Gale (Ed), Bronze Age Trade in the Mediterranean. Göteborg, Paul Åströms Förlag 90, pp 351-386

Simmons, A. 1994. Early Neolithic Settlement in Western Cyprus: Preliminary Report on the 1992-1993 Test Excavations at Kholetria Ortos. *Bulletin of the American School of Oriental Research*, Vol 295, pp 1-14

Sjøvold, T. 1973 The occurance of minor non-metrical variants in the skeleton and their quantitative treatment for population comparisons. *HOMO*, 24:204:233

Sjøvold, T. 1976-1977. A method for familial studies based on minor skeletal variants. *OSSA*, 3/4:97-107.

Sjøvold, T. 1984. A report on the heretibility of some cranial measurements and non-metric traits. In GN van Vark and WW Howells (eds.):*Multivariate statistical methods in physical anthropology*. D. Reidel Publishing Company, pp. 223-246.

Smith, B.H. 1991. Standards of human tooth formation and dental age assessment. In MA Kelley and CS Larsen (eds.): *Advances in Dental Anthropology*. New York: Wiley-Liss, pp 143-168.

Sofaer, J.A., Niswander, J.D., MacLean, C.J. and Workman, P.L. 1972. Population Studies on Southwestern Indian Tribes:V. Tooth morphology as an indicator of biological distance. *American Journal of Physical Anthropology*, 37:357-366

Stanley Price, N.P. 1977a. Khirokitia and the initial settlement of Cyprus. *Levant*, 9:66-89

Stanley Price, N.P. 1977b. Colonization and Continuity in the Early Prehistory of Cyprus. *World Archaeology*, 9(1):27-41

Stanley Price, N.P. 1980. Early Prehistoric Settlement in Cyprus A Review and Gazetteer of Sites, c. 6500-3000 BC. BAR International Series Vol 65.

Stanley Price, N.P. and Christou, D. 1973. Excavations at Khirokitia. *Report of the Department of Antiquities Cyprus*, pp 1-33.

Steele, D.G. 1970. Estimation of stature from fragments of long limb bones. In (ed) TD Stewart, *Personal identification in mass disaster*. National Museum of Natural History, Washington, pp 85-97.

Steele, D.G. and McKern, T.W. 1969. A method for assessment of maximum long bone length and living stature from fragmentary long bones. *American Journal of Physical Anthropology* 31:215-228.

Stone, A.C. 2000. Ancient DNA from skeletal remains. In: M. A. Katzenberg and S. Saunders (eds.), *Biological Anthropology of the Human Skeleton*. New York: Wiley Liss, Inc., pp. 351-371

Stringer, C.B., L.T. Humphrey and T. Compton 1997. Cladistic analysis of dental traits in recent humans using a fossil outgroup. *Journal of Human Evolution*, 32:389-402.

Sutherland, L.D. and Suchey, J.M. 1991. Use of the ventral arch in public sex determination. *Journal of Forensic Sciences*, 36:501-511.

Swiny, S. 1986. The Philia culture and its Foreign relations. In, Karageorghis, V. (ed.) Acts of the International Archaeological Symposium 'Cyprus between the Orient and the Occident'. Zavallis Press, Nicosia, pp 29-44

Todd, I.A. 1986. The Foreign Relations of Cyprus in the Neolithic/Chalcolithic Periods: New evidence from the Vasilikos Valley. In, Vassos Karageorghis (ed.): Acts of the International Archaeological Symposium 'Cyprus between the Orient and the Occident'. Zavallis Press, Nicosia, pp 12-28

Todd, I.A. 1989. Early prehistoric society: a view from the Vasilikos valley. In E Peltenburg (ed.):*Early Society in Cyprus*. University of Edinburgh Press pp. 2-13.

Torgersen, J. 1951. The developmental genetics and evolutionary meaning of the metopic suture. *American Journal of Physical Anthropology* 9:193-210.

Triantaphyllou, S. 1998. Prehistoric cemetery populations from northern Greece: A breath of life for the skeletal remains. In, Keith Branigan (ed.): *Cemetery and Society in the Aegean Bronze Age*. Sheffield Studies in Aegean Archaeology, 1. Sheffield Academic Press, Sheffield, pp 150-164.

Triantaphyllou, S. 2001. A bioarchaeological approach to Prehistoric cemetery populations from Central and Western Greek Macedonia. BAR International Series, 976.

Trinkaus, E. 1978. Bilateral asymmetry on human skeletal non-metric traits. *American Journal of Physical Anthropology*, 49:315-318.

Trotter, M. 1970. Estimation of stature from intact long limb bones. In T.D. Stewart (ed.) *Personal identification in mass disasters*. National Museum of Natural History, Washington, pp. 71-84

Trotter, M. and Gleser, G.C. 1952. Estimation from long bones of American whites and Negroes. *American Journal of Physical Anthropology*, 10:463-514

Turner II, C.G. 1976. Dental evidence on the origins of the Ainu and Japanese. *Science*, 193:911-913

Turner II, C.G. 1979. Dental anthropological indications of agriculture among the Jomon people of central Japan: X. Peopling of the Pacific. *American Journal of Physical Anthropology*, 51:619-635

Turner II, C.G. 1985. The dental search for Native American Origins. In: R. Kirk and E. Szathmary (eds.), Out of Asia: Peopling the Americas and the Pacific. The Journal of Pacific History, Canberra, pp 31-78

Turner II, C.G. 1986. Dentochronogical separation estimates for Pacific Rim populations. *Science*, 232:1140-1142.

Turner II, C.G. 1987. Late Pleistocene and Holocene population history of East Asia based on dental variation. *American Journal of Physical Anthropology*, 73:305-321.

Turner II, C.G. 1992. The Dental Bridge between Australia and Asia: following Macintosh into East Asian hearth of humanity. *Archaeology in Oceania*, 27(3):143-152.

Turner II, C.G. and Markowitz, M.A. 1990. Dental discontinuity between Late Pleistocene and recent Nubians: Peopling of the Eurafrican-South Asian triangle I. *Homo*, 41:32-41.

Turner II, C.G., Nichol, C.R. and Scott, G.R. 1991. Scoring procedure for key morphological traits of the permanent dentition: The Arizona State University Dental Anthropology System. In, M.A. Kelly and C.S. Larsen (eds.), Advances in Dental Anthropology. Wiley-Liss, New York, pp 13-31.

Turner II, C.G. and Swindler, D.R. 1978. The dentition of New Britain West Nakanai Melanesians. *American Journal of Physical Anthropology*, 49:361-372.

Tylecote, R.F. 1981. Chalcolithic metallurgy in the Eastern Mediteranean. In: J. Reade (ed.), Chalcolithic Cyprus and Western Asia. British Museum, Occasional Papers No. 26, pp 41-52

Tyrell, A.J. 2000. Skeletal Non-Metric traits and the assessment of inter- and intra-population diversity: past problems and future potential. In, M. Cox and S. Mays (eds), *Human Osteology in Archaeology and Forensic Science*. Greenwich Medical Media Ltd, pp 289-306.

Tyrrell, A.J. and Chamberlain, A.T. 1998. Non-metric trait evidence for modern human affinities and the distinctiveness of Neaderthals. *Journal of Human Evolution*, 34:549-554.

Ubelaker, D.H. 1978. *Human skeletal remains: Excavation, analysis, interpretation*. Chicago: Aldine.

Ubelaker, D.H. 1989. *Human Skeletal Remains*, 2nd edition. Taraxacum, Washington

Vagnetti, L. 1980. Figurines and Minor Objects from a Chalcolithic Cemetery at Souskiou-Vathyrkakas (Cyprus). *Studi Micenei ed egeo-anatolici*, 72(21):17-72

Vigne, J-D., Carrère, I., Saliége, J-F., Person, A., Bcherens, H., Guilaine, J. and Briois, J.F. 2000a. Predomestic cattle, sheep, goat and pig during the late 9th and the 8th millennium Cal. BC on Cyprus: Preliminary results of Shillourokambos (Parekklisha, Limassol) In, M. Mashkour, A.M. Choyke, H. Buitenhuis and F. Poplin (eds.): Archaeozoology of the Near East IV A: Proceedings of the fourth international symposium on the archaeozoology of southwestern Asia and adjacent areas. ARC Publicatie 32 Groningen, The Netherlands, pp 83-106

Vigne, J-D., Buitenhuis, H. and Davis, S. 2000b. Les premiers pas de la domestication animale à l' ouest de l' Euphrate Chypre et L'Anatolie centrale. *Paléorient*, 25(2):49-62

Washburn, S.L. 1948. Sex differences in the public bone. *American Journal of Physical Anthropology*, 6:199-208.

Watkins, T. 1981. The Chalcolithic period in Cyprus: the background to current research. In: Reade, J. (ed.), Chalcolithic Cyprus and Western Asia. British Museum, Occasional Papers No. 26, pp 9-20

Wenicke, M.H. 1989. Change in Early Helladic II. *American Journal of Archaeology*, 93:495-509

Wijsman, E.M. & Neves, W.A. 1986. The use of nonmetric variation in estimating human population admixture: A test case with Brazilian Blacks, Whites, and Mulatos. *American Journal of Physical Anthropology*, 70: 395-405.

Woolley, L. 1921. Carchemish II. The Town Defences. London.

Wright, S. 1951. The genetical structure of populations. *Ann. Eugenics*, 15:323-354

Yang, D.Y., Eng, B., Waye, J.S., Dudar, J.C. and Saunders, S.R. 1998. Improved DNA extraction from ancient bones using silica-based spin columns. *American Journal of Physical Anthropology*, 105(4):539-543

APPENDIX 1

CHRONOLOGY TABLE OF ALL REGIONS

Time Years BC	Greece Period	LER	AS	Cyprus Period	KM	LL	SOU	AI	EN	Syria Period	JT
1000				LC III					LC IIIB	IRON IIA	
									LC IIIA	IRON IB	
										IRON IA	
				LC II				LC IIB		LB IIA-B	
	LH IIB, IIIA1							LC IIA			
1500										LB I	
	LH I, II A			LC I				LC IA			
				MB III				MC IIIC	MC III	MB IIB-C	
	MH	LER V	AS	MB II							
				MB I						MB IIA	
2000				EB III						MB I	
	EH III			EB II							
		LER IV								EB IV	
	EH II			EB I							
					Period 5						
2500		LER III		Chal III	Period 4	Period 3				EB III	
					Period 3B	Period 2				EB II	Period 2
3000	EH I						Chal II				
				Chal II		Period 1				EB I	
					Period 3A						
3500	LN										
				Chal I	Period 2					Chalcolithic	

Samples included in the present study in a regional chronology. Shaded areas represent approximate time periods from where the human remains are derived (Greek chronology modified from Dickinson 1995 fig 1.3, Cypriot chronology modified from Peltenburg 1989 pp xvi, Syrian chronology modified from Peltenburg et al. 1995 fig 1).

APPENDIX 2

CHRONOLOGY OF CYPRUS

Cypro-PPNB			7000-6000
Neolithic I	Khirokitia		6000-5200
Neolithic II	Sotira		4500-3800
Chalcolithic	Erimi	Early	3800-3500
		Middle	3500-2800
		Late	2800-2300
Early Bronze Age		I	2300-2075
(or Early Cypriot)		II	2075-2000
		III	2000-1900
Middle Bronze Age		I	1900-1800
(or Middle Cypriot)		II	1800-1725
		III	1725-1650
Late Bronze Age		IA	1650-1575
(or Late Cypriot)		IB	1575-1475
		IIA	1475-1400
		IIB	1400-1325
		IIC	1325-1225
		IIIA	1225-1190
		IIIB	1190-1150
		IIIC	1150-1050

All dates are uncalibrated dates B.C. and is only a general guide. Cypro-PPNB (Peltenburg et al. 2001) Neolithic and Bronze Age (Peltenburg 1989:xvi).

APPENDIX 3

CRANIAL NON-METRIC TRAIT FREQUENCIES

Country	Cyprus														
Site	SOU			LL			KM			AI			EN		
Traits	P	n	nt	p	n	nt	p	n	nt	p	n	nt	p	n	nt
Ossicle at lambda	0.00	10	0	-	0	0	0.00	11	0	0.10	21	2	0.09	58	5
Ossicle(s) in lambdoid suture	0.00	10	0	-	0	0	0.00	11	0	0.90	21	19	0.83	58	48
Parietal foramen	0.00	12	0	-	0	0	0.00	18	0	0.49	47	23	0.28	109	30
Ossicle(s) at bregma	0.00	4	0	0.00	14	0	0.00	13	0	0.00	21	0	0.02	57	1
Metopic suture	0.25	4	1	0.11	9	1	0.00	13	0	0.10	21	2	0.09	57	5
Ossicle(s) in coronal suture	0.00	12	0	-	0	0	0.00	18	0	0.00	47	0	0.03	109	3
Bridging of supraorbital notch	0.00	4	0	0.00	14	0	0.00	13	0	0.38	21	8	0.40	57	23
Accessory supraorbital foramen	0.00	4	0	0.00	21	0	0.00	13	0	0.00	21	0	0.00	57	0

Cranial Non-Metric trait frequencies (p = frequency, n = number of bones/teeth, nt = number of bones/teeth with trait)

Country	Greece						Syria		
Site	AS			LER			JT		
Traits	p	n	nt	p	n	nt	p	n	nt
Ossicle at lambda	0	1	0	0	44	0	0	11	0
Ossicle(s) in lambdoid suture	1	1	1	0.07	44	3	0.09	11	1
Parietal foramen	0	2	0	0	87	0	0	22	0
Ossicle(s) at bregma	0	1	0	0	48	0	0	16	0
Metopic suture	0	1	0	0.08	48	4	0.13	16	2
Ossicle(s) in coronal suture	-	0	0	0	87	0	0	22	0
Bridging of supraorbital notch	1	1	1	0.1	48	5	0.13	16	2
Accessory supraorbital foramen	0	1	0	0.1	48	5	0.13	16	2

Cranial Non-Metric trait frequencies (cont...) (p = frequency, n = number of bones/teeth, nt = number of bones/teeth with trait)

APPENDIX 4

POST-CRANIAL NON-METRIC TRAIT FREQUENCIES

Country		Cyprus														
Site		SOU			LL			KM			AI			EN		
Traits	Bone	p	n	nt	p	n	nt	P	n	nt	p	n	nt	p	n	nt
Poirier's facet	Femur	0	4	0	0	5	0	0	12	0	-	0	0	0.4	27	11
Plaque	Femur	0	4	0	0	5	0	0	12	0	-	0	0	0.2	27	6
Medial tibial squatting facet	Tibia	-	0	0	1	1	1	0.3	4	1	-	0	0	-	0	0
Lateral tibial squatting facet	Tibia	-	0	0	1	1	1	0.3	4	1	-	0	0	-	0	0
Septal aperture	Humerus	0.14	14	2	0.6	7	4	0.4	9	4	-	0	0	-	0	0
Vastus notch	Patella	0.25	4	1	0	1	0	0	9	0	-	0	0	-	0	0
Os trigonum	Talus	0	5	0	0	4	0	0	10	0	-	0	0	-	0	0
Medial talar facet	Talus	0	5	0	0	4	0	0	10	0	-	0	0	-	0	0
Lateral talar extension	Talus	0.2	5	1	0	4	0	0	10	0	-	0	0	-	0	0
Double inferior anterior talar facet	Talus	0	5	0	0	4	0	0	10	0	-	0	0	-	0	0
Double anterior calcaneal facet	Calaneus	-	0	0	1	1	1	0.1	7	1	-	0	0	-	0	0
Absent anterior calcaneal facet	Calaneus	-	0	0	0	1	0	0	7	0	-	0	0	-	0	0

Post-Cranial Non-Metric trait frequencies (p = frequency, n = number of bones/teeth, nt = number of bones/teeth with trait)

Country		Greece						Syria		
Site		AS			LER			JT		
Traits	Bone	p	n	Nt	p	n	nt	p	n	nt
Poirier's facet	Femur	0.33	3	1	0.47	49	23	0.42	24	10
Plaque	Femur	0	2	0	0.1	49	5	0.08	24	2
Medial tibial squatting facet	Tibia	0.25	4	1	0.25	60	15	0.4	15	6
Lateral tibial squatting facet	Tibia	0.75	4	3	0.72	60	43	0.47	15	7
Septal aperture	Humerus	0.44	9	4	0.17	114	19	0.41	32	13
Vastus notch	Patella	0.17	6	1	0.18	66	12	0.21	24	5
Os trigonum	Talus	0	5	0	0.17	88	15	0.05	21	1
Medial talar facet	Talus	0	4	0	0.09	88	8	0	22	0
Lateral talar extension	Talus	0	5	0	0	88	0	0.05	22	1
Double inferior anterior talar facet	Talus	0	4	0	0.5	88	44	0.05	22	1
Double anterior calcaneal facet	Calaneus	0.25	4	1	0.54	74	40	0.17	18	3
Absent anterior calcaneal facet	Calaneus	0	4	0	0.05	74	4	0.06	18	1

Post-Cranial Non-Metric trait frequencies (cont...) (p = frequency, n = number of bones/teeth, nt = number of bones/teeth with trait)

APPENDIX 5

DENTAL NON-METRIC TRAIT FREQUENCIES

Country			Cyprus												
Site			SOU			LL			KM			AI			EN		
Traits	Tooth	Range	p	n	nt	p	n	nt	p	n	nt	p	n	nt	p	n	nt
Shoveling	I^1	(2-7)	0.11	19	2	0.18	38	7	0.52	48	25	0.43	7	3	0.33	12	4
	I^2	(2-7)	0.24	17	4	0.28	25	7	0.41	37	15	0.67	12	8	0.43	14	6
	C^1	(2-7)	0.00	12	0	0.16	32	5	0.00	45	0	0.56	9	5	0.55	20	11
	I_1	(2-7)	0.00	24	0	0.04	28	1	0.06	33	2	0.00	1	0	0.00	6	0
	I_2	(2-7)	0.00	14	0	0.00	26	0	0.10	20	2	0.00	0	0	0.50	4	2
Labial convexity	I^1	(2-4)	0.26	19	5	0.00	37	0	0.00	47	0	0.00	7	0	0.00	12	0
	I^2	(2-4)	0.24	17	4	0.00	25	0	0.00	37	0	0.00	12	0	0.00	14	0
Double shoveling	I^1	(2-6)	0.00	19	0	0.00	38	0	0.00	47	0	0.00	7	0	0.00	12	0
	I^2	(2-6)	0.00	17	0	0.00	25	0	0.00	37	0	0.00	12	0	0.00	14	0
	C^1	(2-6)	0.00	12	0	0.00	33	0	0.00	39	0	0.11	9	1	0.00	20	0
	P^3	(2-6)	0.00	15	0	0.00	26	0	0.00	37	0	0.14	14	2	0.12	25	3
	I_1	(2-6)	0.00	24	0	0.00	28	0	0.00	32	0	0.00	1	0	0.00	6	0
	I_2	(2-6)	0.00	14	0	0.00	26	0	0.00	20	0	0.00	0	0	0.00	4	0
Interruption groove	I^1	Present	0.00	19	0	0.05	38	2	0.02	47	1	0.00	7	0	0.00	12	0
	I^2	Present	0.18	17	3	0.20	25	5	0.16	37	6	0.50	12	6	0.00	14	0
Tuberculum dentale	I^1	(2-6)	0.11	19	2	0.24	33	8	0.26	47	12	0.00	7	0	0.00	12	0
	I^2	(2-6)	0.24	17	4	0.20	25	5	0.24	37	9	0.00	12	0	0.14	14	2
	C^1	(2-6)	0.00	12	0	0.18	33	6	0.28	39	11	0.11	9	1	0.50	20	10
Canine mesial ridge	C^1	(2-3)	0.00	12	0	0.00	33	0	0.00	45	0	0.00	9	0	0.25	20	5
Canine distal accessory ridge	C^1	(2-5)	0.00	12	0	0.30	33	10	0.03	39	1	0.00	9	0	0.00	20	0
	C_1	(2-5)	0.00	28	0	0.25	20	5	0.00	26	0	0.00	1	0	0.00	4	0
PM mesial & distal accessory cusps	P^3	1	0.00	15	0	0.00	26	0	0.00	37	0	0.00	14	0	0.00	25	0
	P^4	1	0.00	26	0	0.00	23	0	0.00	36	0	0.00	14	0	0.00	22	0
Tricuspid premolars	P^3	1	0.00	15	0	0.00	26	0	0.00	37	0	0.00	14	0	0.00	25	0
	P^4	1	0.00	26	0	0.00	23	0	0.00	36	0	0.00	14	0	0.00	22	0
Distosagittal ridge	P^3	1	0.00	15	0	0.00	26	0	0.00	40	0	0.00	14	0	0.00	25	0
Metacone expression	M^1	(3-5)	1.00	10	10	1.00	35	35	1.00	42	42	0.96	24	23	1.00	32	32
	M^2	(3-5)	1.00	7	7	1.00	27	27	0.91	32	29	0.96	27	26	1.00	32	32
	M^3	(3-5)	0.83	6	5	0.80	10	8	0.94	18	17	1.00	13	13	0.96	28	27
Hypocone expression	M^1	(3-5)	0.80	10	8	1.00	35	35	1.00	42	42	0.96	24	23	1.00	32	32
	M^2	(3-5)	0.86	7	6	0.56	27	15	0.39	28	11	0.81	27	22	0.84	32	27
	M^3	(3-5)	0.00	6	0	0.50	10	5	0.17	18	3	0.15	13	2	0.39	28	11
Cusp 5	M^1	(2-5)	0.00	8	0	0.06	35	2	0.13	40	5	0.00	24	0	0.00	32	0
	M^2	(2-5)	0.14	7	1	0.11	27	3	0.10	29	3	0.00	27	0	0.00	32	0
	M^3	(2-5)	0.00	6	0	0.10	10	1	0.06	18	1	0.15	13	2	0.00	28	0
Carabelli trait	M^1	(2-7)	0.00	8	0	0.37	35	13	0.24	42	10	0.21	24	5	0.06	32	2
	M^2	(2-7)	0.00	7	0	0.00	27	0	0.00	29	0	0.07	27	2	0.00	32	0
	M^3	(2-7)	0.17	6	1	0.00	10	0	0.00	20	0	0.00	13	0	0.00	28	0
Parastyle	M^1	(2-6)	0.00	8	0	0.00	35	0	0.00	42	0	0.00	23	0	0.00	32	0
	M^2	(2-6)	0.14	7	1	0.00	27	0	0.00	33	0	0.00	27	0	0.00	32	0
	M^3	(2-6)	0.00	6	0	0.00	10	0	0.00	20	0	0.00	13	0	0.00	28	0

Dental Non-Metric trait frequencies (p = frequency, n = number of bones/teeth, nt = number of bones/teeth with trait)

APPENDIX 5

DENTAL NON-METRIC TRAIT FREQUENCIES (cont...)

Country			Cyprus														
Site			SOU			LL			KM			AI			EN		
Traits	Tooth	Range	p	n	nt	p	n	nt	p	n	nt	p	n	nt	p	n	nt
Enamel extension	P^3	(2-3)	0.00	15	0	0.00	26	0	0.00	32	0	0.00	14	0	0.00	25	0
	P^4	(2-3)	0.00	26	0	0.00	23	0	0.00	33	0	0.00	14	0	0.00	22	0
	M^1	(2-3)	0.00	8	0	0.00	35	0	0.00	39	0	0.00	23	0	0.00	32	0
	M^2	(2-3)	0.00	7	0	0.00	27	0	0.00	33	0	0.00	27	0	0.00	32	0
	M^3	(2-3)	0.00	6	0	0.00	10	0	0.00	20	0	0.00	13	0	0.00	28	0
Upper premolar root number	P^3	(2-3)	0.00	15	0	0.25	24	6	0.11	28	3	0.00	14	0	0.00	25	0
	P^4	(2-3)	0.00	26	0	0.19	21	4	0.00	30	0	0.00	14	0	0.00	22	0
Peg shaped lateral incisor	I^1	(1-2)	0.00	19	0	0.00	43	0	0.00	54	0	0.00	7	0	0.00	12	0
Peg shaped third molar	M^3	(1-2)	0.00	24	0	0.00	10	0	0.00	20	0	0.00	13	0	0.00	28	0
Odontome	P^3	1	0.00	15	0	0.00	26	0	0.00	40	0	0.00	14	0	0.00	25	0
	P^4	1	0.00	26	0	0.00	23	0	0.00	38	0	0.00	14	0	0.00	22	0
	P_3	1	0.00	29	0	0.00	19	0	0.00	15	0	-	0	0	0.00	5	0
	P_4	1	0.00	21	0	0.00	11	0	0.00	12	0	-	0	0	0.00	3	0
Lower premolar lingual cusps	P_3	(2-9)	0.00	29	0	0.47	19	9	0.36	14	5	-	0	0	1.00	5	5
	P_4	(2-9)	0.00	21	0	0.09	11	1	0.42	12	5	-	0	0	1.00	3	3
Lower molar groove pattern	M_1	Y	0.95	19	18	0.74	23	17	0.81	27	22	1.00	1	1	0.67	6	4
	M_1	+	0.00	19	0	0.26	23	6	0.15	27	4	0.00	1	0	0.33	6	2
	M_1	X	0.00	19	0	0.00	23	0	0.04	27	1	0.00	1	0	0.00	6	0
	M_2	Y	0.14	21	3	0.07	14	1	0.00	23	0	0.25	4	1	0.00	8	0
	M_2	+	0.81	21	17	0.79	14	11	0.96	23	22	0.75	4	3	0.88	8	7
	M_2	X	0.05	21	1	0.14	14	2	0.00	23	0	0.00	4	0	0.13	8	1
	M_3	Y	0.71	7	5	0.14	7	1	0.50	8	4	1.00	1	1	0.00	2	0
	M_3	+	0.29	7	2	0.71	7	5	0.50	8	4	0.00	1	0	1.00	2	2
	M_3	X	0.00	7	0	0.14	7	1	0.00	8	0	0.00	1	0	0.00	2	0
Deflecting wrinkle	M_1	(2-3)	0.00	28	0	0.39	23	9	0.26	27	7	0.00	1	0	0.00	6	0
Distal trigonid crest	M_1	1	0.00	28	0	0.00	23	0	0.00	34	0	0.00	1	0	0.00	6	0
	M_2	1	0.00	41	0	0.00	15	0	0.00	23	0	0.00	4	0	0.00	8	0
	M_3	1	0.00	17	0	0.00	7	0	0.00	8	0	0.00	1	0	0.00	2	0
Protostylid	M_1	(2-7)	0.00	28	0	0.00	23	0	0.00	27	0	0.00	1	0	0.00	6	0
	M_2	(2-7)	0.00	41	0	0.00	15	0	0.00	26	0	0.00	4	0	0.00	8	0
	M_3	(2-7)	0.00	17	0	0.00	7	0	0.00	8	0	0.00	1	0	0.00	2	0
Cusp 5 (hypocunulid)	M_1	(2-5)	0.53	19	10	0.43	23	10	0.40	25	10	1.00	1	1	0.67	6	4
	M_2	(2-5)	0.10	21	2	0.07	14	1	0.00	23	0	0.25	4	1	0.00	8	0
	M_3	(2-5)	0.43	7	3	0.00	7	0	0.38	8	3	1.00	1	1	0.00	2	0

Dental Non-Metric trait frequencies (cont...) (p = frequency, n = number of bones/teeth, nt = number of bones/teeth with trait)

APPENDIX 5

DENTAL NON-METRIC TRAIT FREQUENCIES (cont...)

Country			Greece						Syria		
Site			AS			LER			JT		
Traits	Tooth	Range	p	n	nt	p	n	nt	p	n	nt
Shoveling	I^1	(2-7)	0.88	8	7	0.35	71	25	0.14	21	3
	I^2	(2-7)	1.00	2	2	0.62	63	39	0.67	18	12
	C^1	(2-7)	0.78	9	7	0.27	81	22	0.58	24	14
	I_1	(2-7)	0.00	5	0	0.01	69	1	0	9	0
	I_2	(2-7)	0.00	10	0	0.01	82	1	0.13	16	2
Labial convexity	I^1	(2-4)	0.00	8	0	0.00	71	0	0.29	21	6
	I^2	(2-4)	0.00	2	0	0.03	63	2	0.11	18	2
Double shoveling	I^1	(2-6)	0.00	8	0	0.00	71	0	0	21	0
	I^2	(2-6)	0.00	2	0	0.00	63	0	0	18	0
	C^1	(2-6)	0.00	9	0	0.00	81	0	0	24	0
	P^3	(2-6)	0.10	10	1	0.00	63	0	0.38	13	5
	I_1	(2-6)	0.00	5	0	0.00	69	0	0	9	0
	I_2	(2-6)	0.00	10	0	0.00	82	0	0	16	0
Interruption groove	I^1	Present	0.00	8	0	0.13	71	9	0.1	21	2
	I^2	Present	0.00	2	0	0.13	63	8	0.22	18	4
Tuberculum dentale	I^1	(2-6)	0.00	8	0	0.08	71	6	0.14	21	3
	I^2	(2-6)	0.00	2	0	0.17	63	11	0.28	18	5
	C^1	(2-6)	0.11	9	1	0.40	78	31	0.5	24	12
Canine mesial ridge	C^1	(2-3)	0.00	9	0	0.00	78	0	0	24	0
Canine distal accessory ridge	C^1	(2-5)	0.00	9	0	0.04	78	3	0	24	0
	C_1	(2-5)	0.11	9	1	0.00	88	0	0.09	22	2
PM mesial & distal accessory cusps	P^3	1	0.00	10	0	0.00	63	0	0	13	0
	P^4	1	0.00	5	0	0.00	68	0	0	10	0
Tricuspid premolars	P^3	1	0.00	10	0	0.00	63	0	0	13	0
	P^4	1	0.00	5	0	0.00	68	0	0	10	0
Distosagittal ridge	P^3	1	0.00	10	0	0.00	63	0	0	13	0
Metacone expression	M^1	(3-5)	1.00	16	16	1.00	100	100	0.92	25	23
	M^2	(3-5)	1.00	5	5	0.99	72	71	1	15	15
	M^3	(3-5)	0.88	8	7	0.95	41	39	0.82	11	9
Hypocone expression	M^1	(3-5)	1.00	16	16	1.00	100	100	0.86	21	18
	M^2	(3-5)	0.80	5	4	0.86	72	62	0.86	14	12
	M^3	(3-5)	0.75	8	6	0.63	41	26	0.2	10	2
Cusp 5	M^1	(2-5)	0.00	16	0	0.00	100	0	0.04	26	1
	M^2	(2-5)	0.00	5	0	0.03	72	2	0	15	0
	M^3	(2-5)	0.13	8	1	0.02	41	1	0	13	0
Carabelli trait	M^1	(2-7)	0.19	16	3	0.34	100	34	0.32	25	8
	M^2	(2-7)	0.00	5	0	0.00	72	0	0.07	15	1
	M^3	(2-7)	0.00	8	0	0.05	41	2	0	13	0
Parastyle	M^1	(2-6)	0.00	16	0	0.00	100	0	0	27	0
	M^2	(2-6)	0.00	5	0	0.00	72	0	0	15	0
	M^3	(2-6)	0.00	8	0	0.00	41	0	0	15	0

Dental Non-Metric trait frequencies (cont...) (p = frequency, n = number of bones/teeth, nt = number of bones/teeth with trait)

APPENDIX 5

DENTAL NON-METRIC TRAIT FREQUENCIES (cont...)

Country			Greece						Syria		
Site			AS			LER			JT		
Traits	Tooth	Range	p	n	nt	p	n	nt	p	n	nt
Enamel extension	P^3	(2-3)	0.00	10	0	0.00	63	0	0	13	0
	P^4	(2-3)	0.00	5	0	0.00	68	0	0	10	0
	M^1	(2-3)	0.00	16	0	0.00	100	0	0	27	0
	M^2	(2-3)	0.00	5	0	0.00	72	0	0.07	14	1
	M^3	(2-3)	0.00	8	0	0.00	41	0	0	15	0
Upper premolar root number	P^3	(2-3)	0.00	9	0	0.05	63	3	0	9	0
	P^4	(2-3)	0.00	5	0	0.00	68	0	0.14	7	1
Peg shaped lateral incisor	I^1	(1-2)	0.00	8	0	0.00	71	0	0	21	0
Peg shaped third molar	M^3	(1-2)	0.00	9	0	0.00	47	0	0	15	0
Odontome	P^3	1	0.00	10	0	0.00	63	0	0	13	0
	P^4	1	0.00	5	0	0.00	68	0	0	11	0
	P_3	1	0.00	13	0	0.00	85	0	0	23	0
	P_4	1	0.00	7	0	0.00	83	0	0	16	0
Lower premolar lingual cusps	P_3	(2-9)	0.77	13	10	0.39	85	33	0	23	0
	P_4	(2-9)	0.71	7	5	0.45	83	37	0	17	0
Lower molar groove pattern	M_1	Y	0.70	27	19	0.75	109	82	0.62	26	16
	M_1	+	0.30	27	8	0.15	109	16	0.15	26	4
	M_1	X	0.00	27	0	0.07	109	8	0.04	26	1
	M_2	Y	0.07	15	1	0.05	82	4	0.26	23	6
	M_2	+	0.87	15	13	0.85	82	70	0.52	23	12
	M_2	X	0.07	15	1	0.10	82	8	0.09	23	4
	M_3	Y	-	0	0	0.17	41	7	0.5	14	2
	M_3	+	-	0	0	0.51	41	21	0.43	14	2
	M_3	X	-	0	0	0.32	41	13	0	14	2
Deflecting wrinkle	M_1	(2-3)	0.22	27	6	0.07	109	8	0.03	29	5
Distal trigonid crest	M_1	1	0.00	27	0	0.00	109	0	0	34	0
	M_2	1	0.00	15	0	0.00	82	0	0	27	0
	M_3	1	-	0	0	0.00	41	0	0	16	0
Protostylid	M_1	(2-7)	0.00	27	0	0.00	109	0	0	34	0
	M_2	(2-7)	0.00	15	0	0.00	82	0	0	27	0
	M_3	(2-7)	-	0	0	0.00	41	0	0	16	0
Cusp 5 (hypocunulid)	M_1	(2-5)	0.67	27	18	0.71	109	77	0.44	27	7
	M_2	(2-5)	0.13	15	2	0.04	82	3	0.26	23	4
	M_3	(2-5)	-	0	0	0.17	41	7	0.36	11	5

Dental Non-Metric trait frequencies (cont...) (p = frequency, n = number of bones/teeth, nt = number of bones/teeth with trait)

APPENDIX 6

DENTAL NON-METRIC TRAIT FREQUENCIES OF COMPARATIVE SAMPLES

Trait	Tooth	Range	EUR nt	EUR p	EUR n	NAF nt	NAF p	NAF n	NAT nt	NAT p	NAT n	EBA nt	EBA p	EBA n
Shoveling	I^1	(2-7)	24	0.17	141	24	0.159	154	6	0.1	59	-	-	-
	I^2	(2-7)	-	-	-	-	-	-	-	-	-	2	0.18	11
Double shoveling	I^1	(2-6)	32	0.233	137	15	0.086	175	12	0.12	100	2	0.167	12
	I^2	(2-6)	-	-	-	-	-	-	-	-	-	-	-	-
Interruption groove	I^1	Present	-	-	-	-	-	-	-	-	-	5	0.5	10
	I^2	Present	-	-	-	75	0.361	208	12	0.13	92	7	0.636	11
Tuberculum dentale	I^1	(2-6)	-	-	-	-	-	-	-	-	-	2	0.167	12
	I^2	(2-6)	58	0.381	152	111	0.587	189	58	0.951	61	2	0.222	9
	C^1	(2-6)	-	-	-	-	-	-	-	-	-	4	0.4	10
Canine distal accessory ridge	C^1	(2-5)	46	0.517	89	68	0.349	195	8	0.364	22	4	0.571	7
	C_1	(2-5)	-	-	-	-	-	-	-	-	-	3	0.3	10
PM mesial & distal accessory cusps	P^3	1	-	-	-	-	-	-	-	-	-	3	0.273	11
	P^4	1	-	-	-	-	-	-	-	-	-	1	0.111	9
Metacone expression	M^1	(3-5)	-	-	-	-	-	-	-	-	-	20	1	20
	M^2	(3-5)	-	-	-	-	-	-	-	-	-	15	1	15
	M^3	(3-5)	-	-	-	-	-	-	-	-	-	12	1	12
Hypocone expression	M^1	(3-5)	-	-	-	-	-	-	-	-	-	17	1	17
	M^2	(3-5)	181	0.794	228	427	0.957	446	134	0.912	147	9	0.818	11
	M^3	(3-5)	-	-	-	-	-	-	-	-	-	7	0.778	9
Cusp 5	M^1	(2-5)	29	0.137	212	66	0.185	357	6	0.032	189	6	0.5	12
Cusp 6	M^2	(2-5)	-	-	-	-	-	-	-	-	-	5	0.556	9
Cusp 7	M^3	(2-5)	-	-	-	-	-	-	-	-	-	4	0.4	10

Dental Non-Metric trait frequencies of comparative samples (cont...) (p = frequency, n = number of bones/teeth, nt = number of bones/teeth with trait) (EUR and NAF from Irish 1998:84, NAT from Irish 2000:400-401, EBA from Cucina et al 1999:406-407)

APPENDIX 6

DENTAL NON-METRIC TRAIT FREQUENCIES OF COMPARATIVE SAMPLES (cont...)

Trait (cont.)	Tooth	Range	EUR			NAF			NAT			EBA		
			Nt	P	N	Nt	p	N	Nt	p	N	Nt	p	N
Carabelli trait	M^1	(2-7)	109	0.474	230	181	0.547	331	73	0.81	90	9	0.692	13
	M^2	(2-7)	-	-	-	-	-	-	-	-	-	1	0.091	11
	M^3	(2-7)	-	-	-	-	-	-	-	-	-	1	0.1	10
Parastyle	M^1	(2-6)	-	-	-	-	-	-	-	-	-	5	0.278	18
	M^2	(2-6)	-	-	-	-	-	-	-	-	-	2	0.154	13
	M^3	(2-6)	6	0.045	134	4	0.012	332	1	0.008	133	2	0.182	11
Enamel extension	M^1	(2-3)	125	0.437	286	34	0.068	503	-	-	-	2	0.118	17
	M^2	(2-3)	-	-	-	-	-	-	-	-	-	3	0.25	12
	M^3	(2-3)	-	-	-	-	-	-	-	-	-	2	0.2	10
Upper PM root number	P^3	(2-3)	-	-	-	-	-	-	-	-	-	5	0.357	14
	P^4	(2-3)	-	-	-	-	-	-	-	-	-	10	0.909	11
Peg shaped third molar	M^3	(1-2)	50	0.207	241	100	0.183	545	-	-	-	-	-	-
Odontome	P^3	1	2	0.012	171	1	0.002	441	1	0.006	161	-	-	-
Lower premolar lingual cusps	P$_3$	(2-9)	100	0.629	159	196	0.726	270	59	0.602	98	5	0.357	14
	P$_4$	(2-9)	-	-	-	-	-	-	-	-	-	7	0.636	11
Lower molar groove pattern	M$_2$	Y	49	0.229	214	123	0.306	402	47	0.305	154	-	-	-
Deflecting wrinkle	M$_1$	(2-3)	46	0.309	149	66	0.247	267	4	0.034	119	10	1	10
Distal trigonid crest	M$_1$	1	16	0.086	185	9	0.033	276	-	-	-	4	0.364	11
	M$_2$	1	-	-	-	-	-	-	-	-	-	1	0.091	11
	M$_3$	1	-	-	-	-	-	-	-	-	-	1	0.2	5
Protostylid	M$_1$	(2-7)	40	0.2	200	114	0.325	351	21	0.144	146	2	0.133	15
	M$_2$	(2-7)	-	-	-	-	-	-	-	-	-	2	0.182	11
	M$_3$	(2-7)	-	-	-	-	-	-	-	-	-	4	0.8	5
Cusp 5 (hypocunulid)	M$_1$	(2-5)	-	-	-	-	-	-	-	-	-	13	0.812	16
Cusp 5 (hypocunulid)	M$_2$	(2-5)	-	-	-	-	-	-	-	-	-	3	0.231	13
Cusp 5 (hypocunulid)	M$_3$	(2-5)	-	-	-	-	-	-	-	-	-	30	5	6

Dental Non-Metric trait frequencies of comparative samples (cont...) (p = frequency, n = number of bones/teeth, nt = number of bones/teeth with trait) (EUR and NAF from Irish 1998:84, NAT from Irish 2000:400-401, EBA from Cucina et al 1999:406-407)

APPENDIX 7

CRANIAL NON-METRIC OF COMPARATIVE SAMPLES

Site	Dynastic Egypt			Lachish			Badari		
Traits	p	n	nt	P	n	nt	p	n	nt
Ossicle at lambda	0.15	55	8	0.11	54	6	0.10	48	5
Ossicle(s) in lambdoid suture	0.25	110	27	0.30	107	32	0.30	96	29
Ossicle(s) at bregma	0.00	105	0	0.00	53	0	0.00	48	0
Ossicle(s) in coronal suture	0.00	110	0	0.04	108	4	0.02	96	2
Parietal foramen	0.56	110	62	0.35	108	38	0.32	96	31
Metopic suture	0.04	55	2	0.07	54	4	0.06	48	3
Bridging of supraorbital notch	0.10	110	11	0.18	108	19	0.15	96	14
Accessory supraorbital foramen	0.39	110	43	0.19	108	20	0.18	96	17

Cranial Non-Metric of comparative samples (p = frequency, n = number of bones/teeth, nt = number of bones/teeth with trait) (Dynastic Egypt from Berry and Berry 1967, Lachish from Risdon 1939 and Berry and Berry 1967, Badari from Morant 1935 and Berry et al. 1967).

APPENDIX 8

EQUATIONS

Glossary for symbols:
n = sample size
N = actual population size
n = absolute frequency of traits
p = relative frequency in the sample size (p = x/n)
P = actual frequency in actual population (P = X/N)

Anscombe transformation (Anscombe 1948)

$$P = \frac{x + 3/8}{n + 3/4}$$

Where p = relative frequency of a trait in the sample, x = absolute frequency of that trait (i.e. the number of indices recorded) and n = sample size (all individuals, or sides)

Mean Measure of Divergence (MMD)

$$MMD = 1/r \sum_{i=1}^{r} [(\theta_{1i} - \theta_{2i})^2 - V_{12i}]$$

Where θ_{1i} is: arcsin $(1-2p1i)$, where p1i denotes the frequency of the ith trait in population 1 and r is the total number of traits studied. V_{12i} is a correction which attempts to ensure that the MMD is independent of sample size. V_{12i} is given as:

$$V_{12i} = (1/n1i + \tfrac{1}{2}) + (1/n2i + \tfrac{1}{2})$$

MMD significance test:

Standard deviation of the MMD = $\sqrt{\text{variance MMD}}$ = $\sqrt{2/r^2 \sum_{i=1}^{r} V_{12i}^2}$

The MMD is regarded as significant if it is more than or equal to twice this expression.

Coefficient of θ (*D.θ*) (Tyrrell & Chamberlain 1998)

If p_x is the frequency of the presence of a trait in population x, then $1- p_x$ is the frequency of the absence of the trait, and the heterogeneity of the trait in population x is:

$$h_x = 2(p_x - p_x^2)$$

For two population samples x and y with respective samples sizes n_x and n_y, the within-population heterogeneity for a single trait is estimated as:

$$b = (n_x \cdot h_x + n_y \cdot h_y) / (n_x + n_y - 1)$$

and the total heterogeneity for a single trait is estimated as:

$$a + b = \frac{[2n_x \cdot (p_x\ 0.5)2 + 2n_y \cdot (p_y\ 0.5)2] + b \cdot (n^* \ 0.5)}{n^*}$$

where $n^* = 2(n_x \cdot n_y) / (n_x + n_y)$

The between-population heterogeneity is estimated as:

$$a = (a + b) - b$$

and the F_{ST} analogue θ is given by:

$$\theta = a / (a+b)$$

The effective genetic distance is then calculated as:

$$D.\theta = -\log_n (1 - \theta)$$

The value D. θ was calculated for each possible pair of populations in the study sample.

Kolmogorov-Smirnov Test

$$1.36 \sqrt{\frac{n_1 + n_2}{n_1 n_2}}$$

Where n_1 = the number of individuals in sample 1 and n_2 = the number of individuals in sample 2. For this example the significance level is set at 0.05. If 0.01 level is required, the coefficient is 1.63; if 0.001 it is 1.95 (Shennan 1997:57).

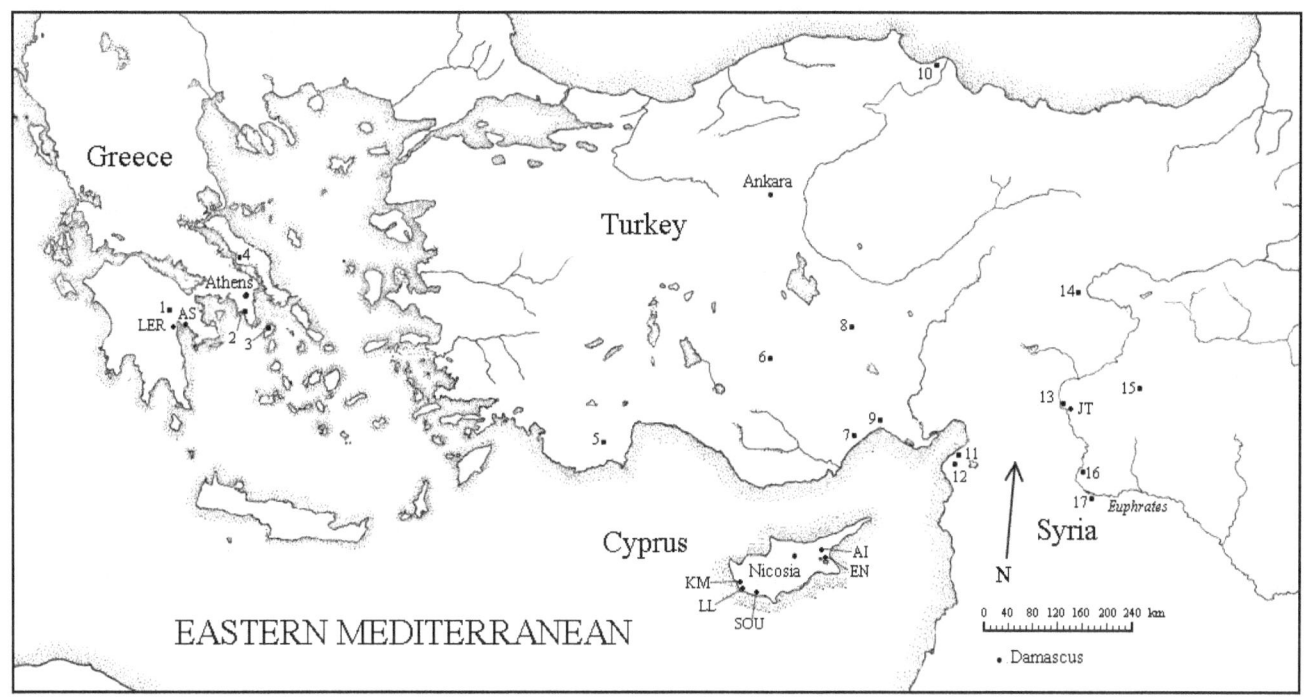

Map 1 – Eastern Mediterranean. All site in this study plus extra sites mentioned in text (Modified from Angel 1971:10).

Greece
1. Mycenae
2. Ayios Kosmas
3. Manika-Chalkis
4. Kephala

Turkey
5. Karataş-Semayük
6. Çatal Hüyük
7. Mersin
8. Çiftlik
9. Tarsus
10. İkiztepe
11. Şeyh Höyük
12. Amuq
13. Carchemish
14. Değimentepe
15. Kurban Höyük

Syria
16. Mureybet
17. Abu Hureyra

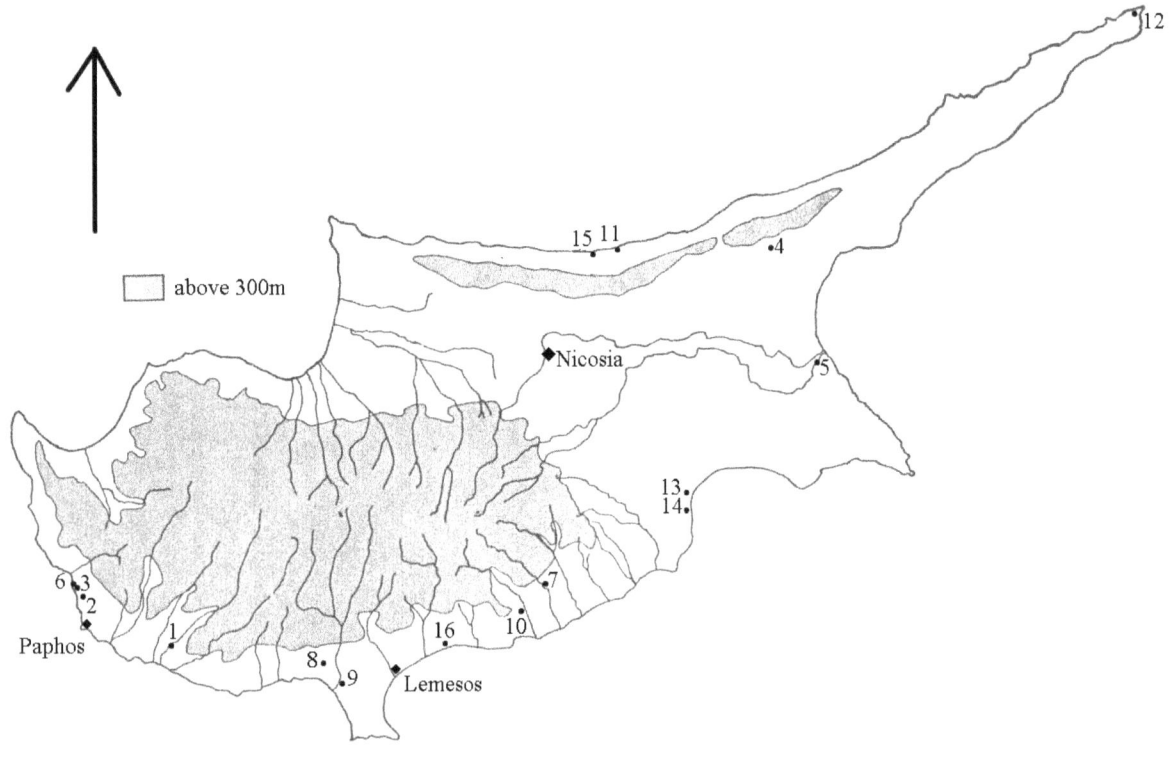

Map 2 – Cyprus. All major sites on Cyprus mentioned in text.

1. Souskiou
2. Lemba-Lakkous
3. Kissonerga-Mosphilia
4. Ayios Iakovos
5. Enkomi
6. Kissonerga-Mylouthkia
7. Khirokitia
8. Sotira
9. Erimi-Pamboula
10. Kalavasos-Tenta
11. Troulli
12. Cape Andreas
13. Kition
14. Hala Sultan Teke
15. Ayios Epiktitos-Vrysi
16. Parekklisha-Shillourokambos

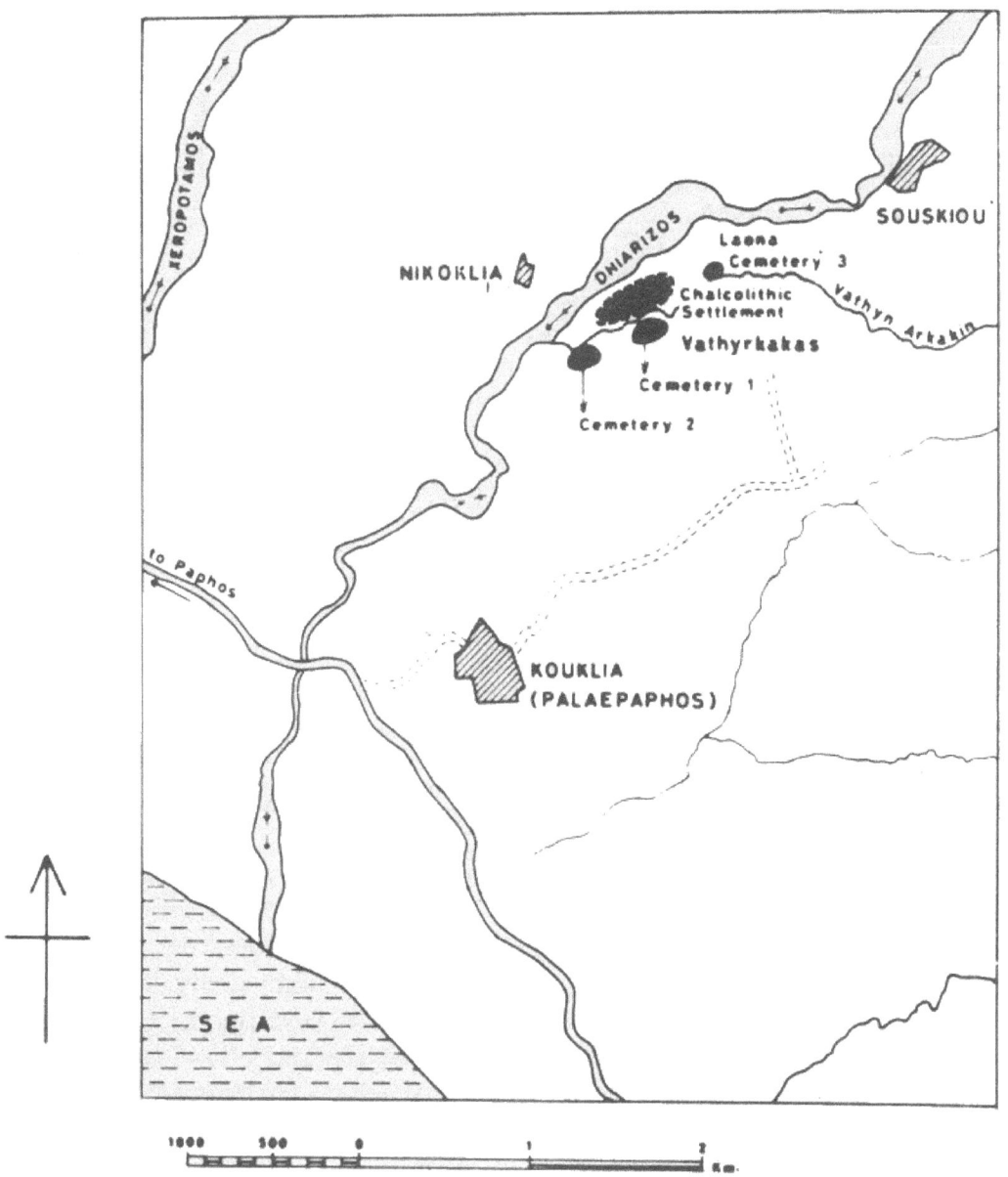

Map 3 – Souskiou general area (Christou 1989:83)

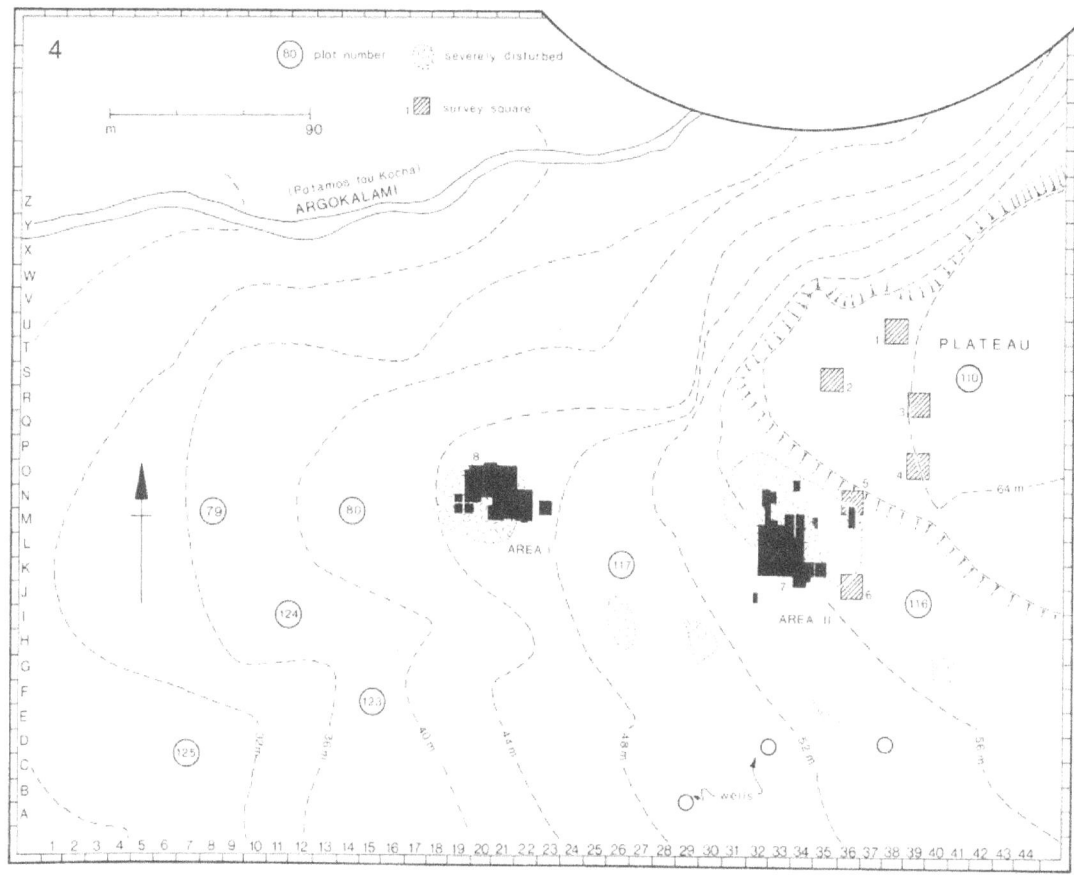

Map 4 – Lemba-Lakkous main area (Peltenburg et al. 1985 fig 7)

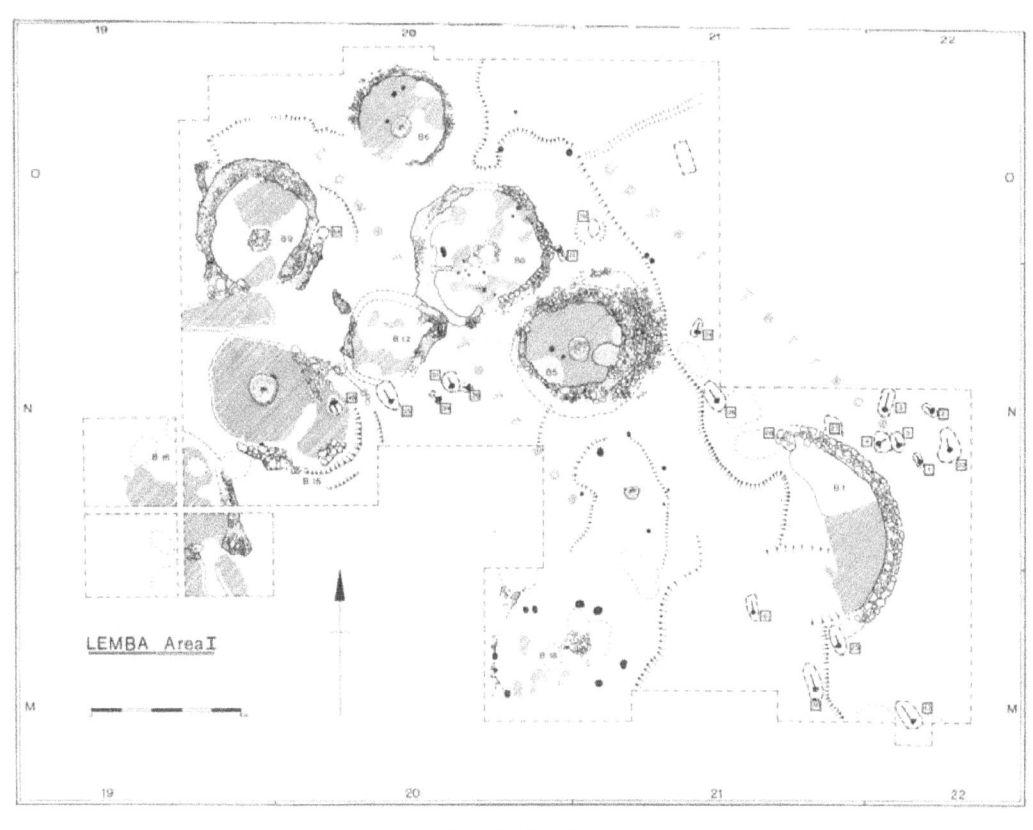

Map – 5 Lemba-Lakkous Area 1 (Peltenburg et al. 1985 fig 10)

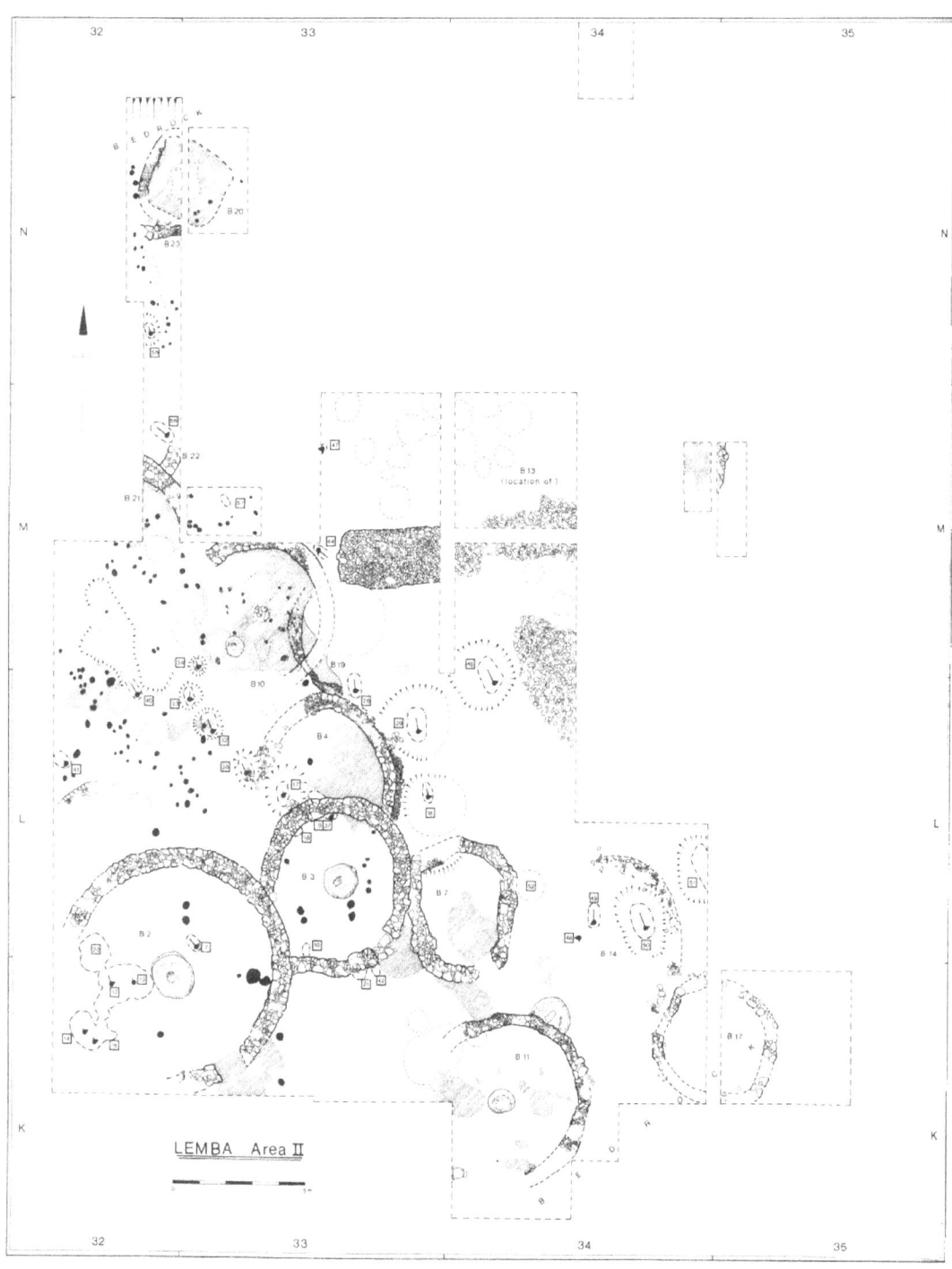

Map 6 – Lemba-Lakkous Area 2 (Peltenburg et al. 1985 fig 22)

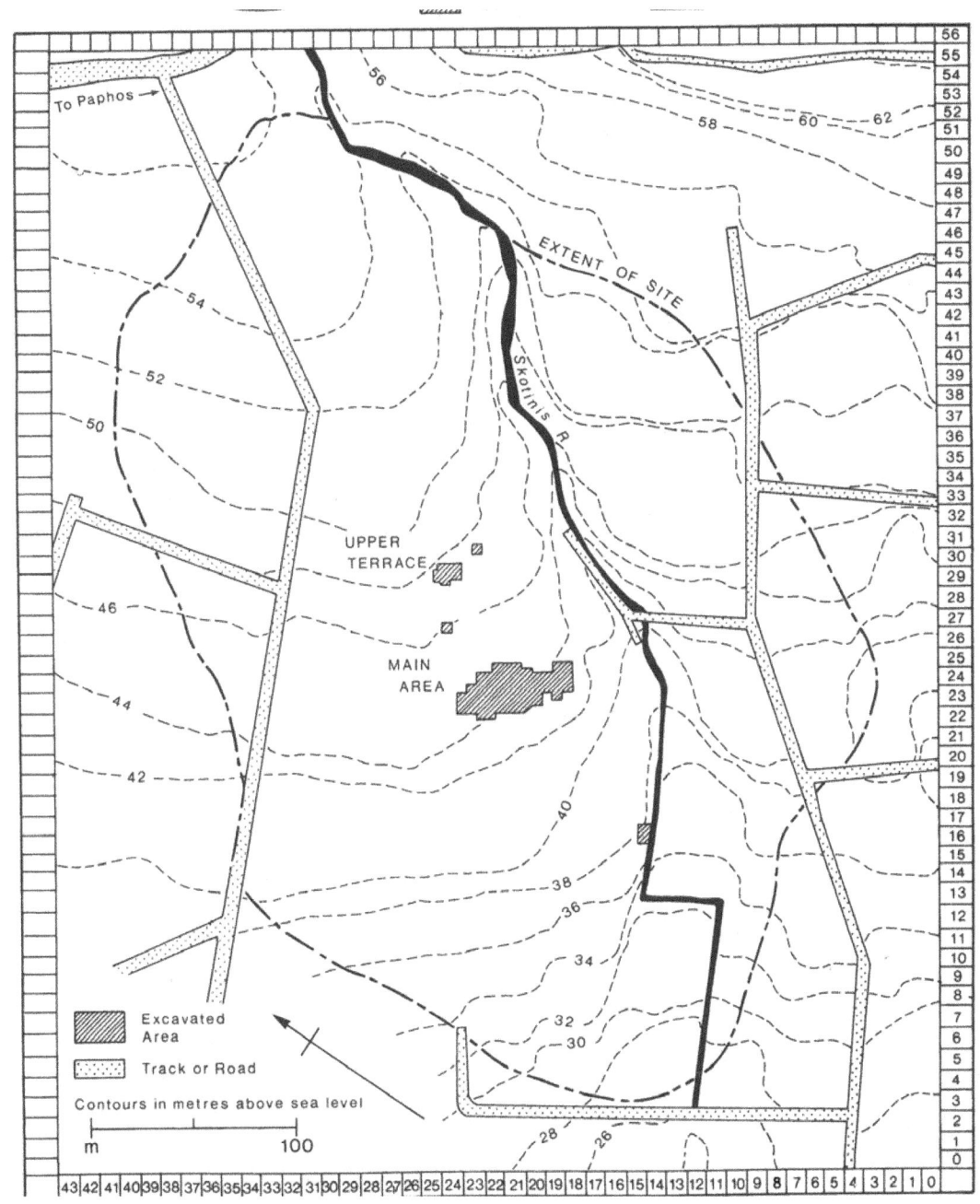

Map 7 – Kissonerga-Mosphilia general area (Peltenburg et al. 1998 fig 15)

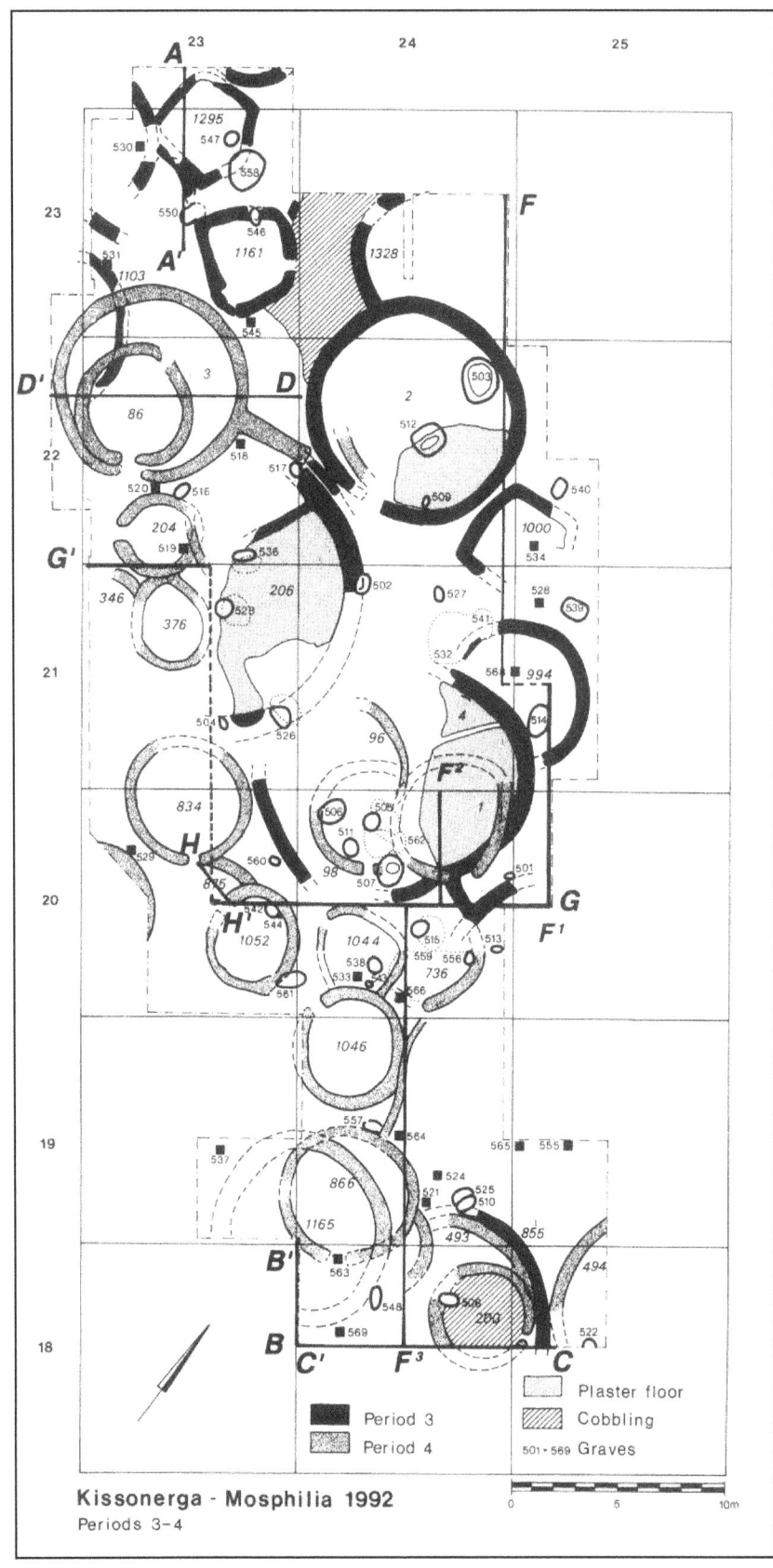

ap 8 – Kissonerga-Mosphilia main area (Peltenburg et al. 1998 fig 17)

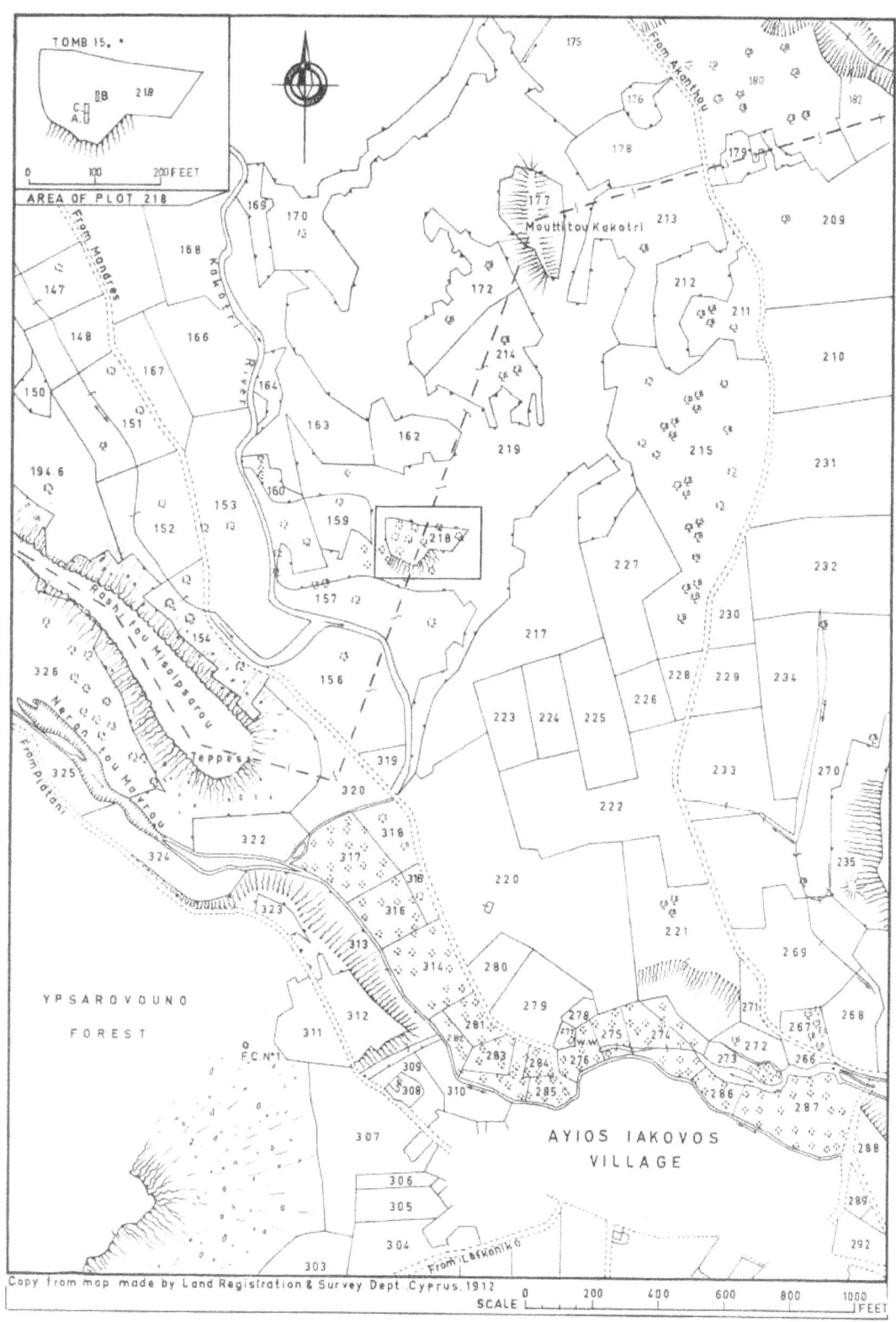

Map 9 – Ayios Iakovos general area (Åström 1969:41).

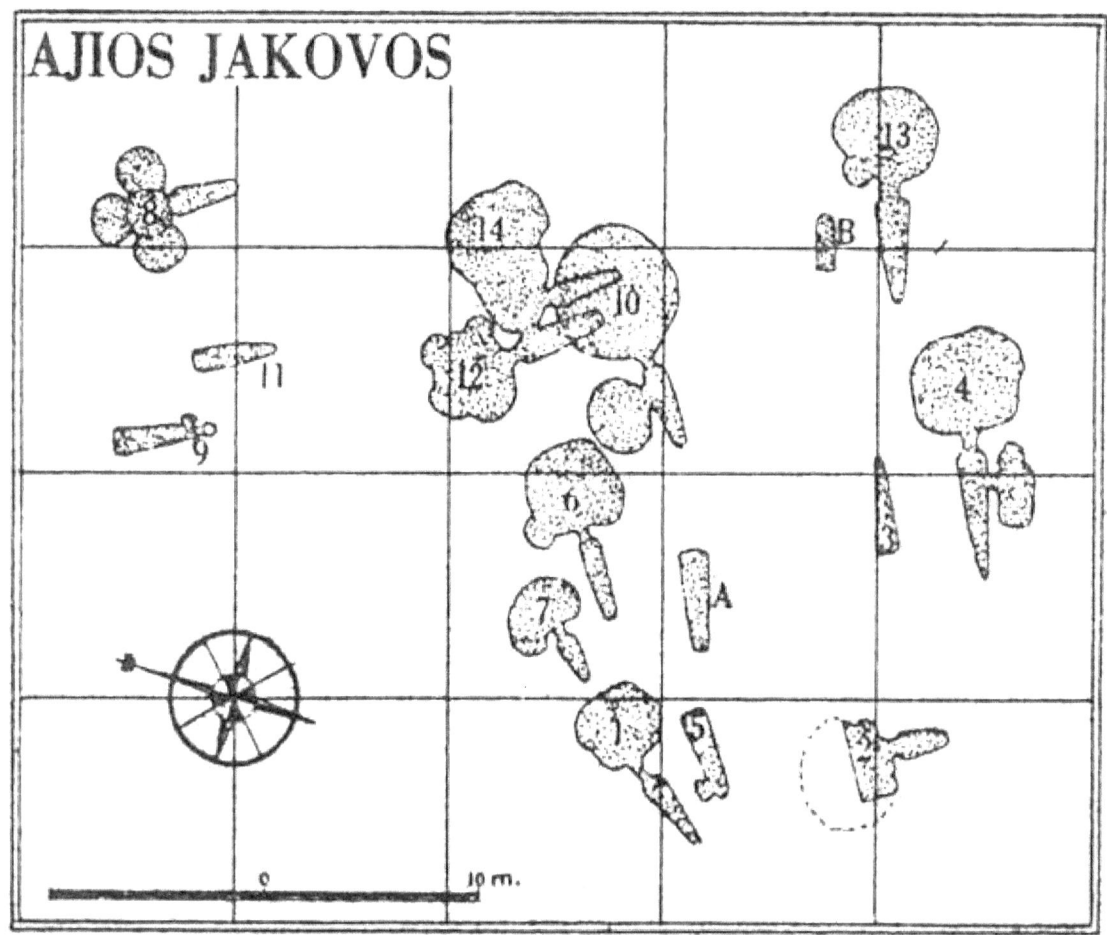

Map 10 – Ayios Iakovos drawings of chamber tombs (Gjerstad et al. 1934).

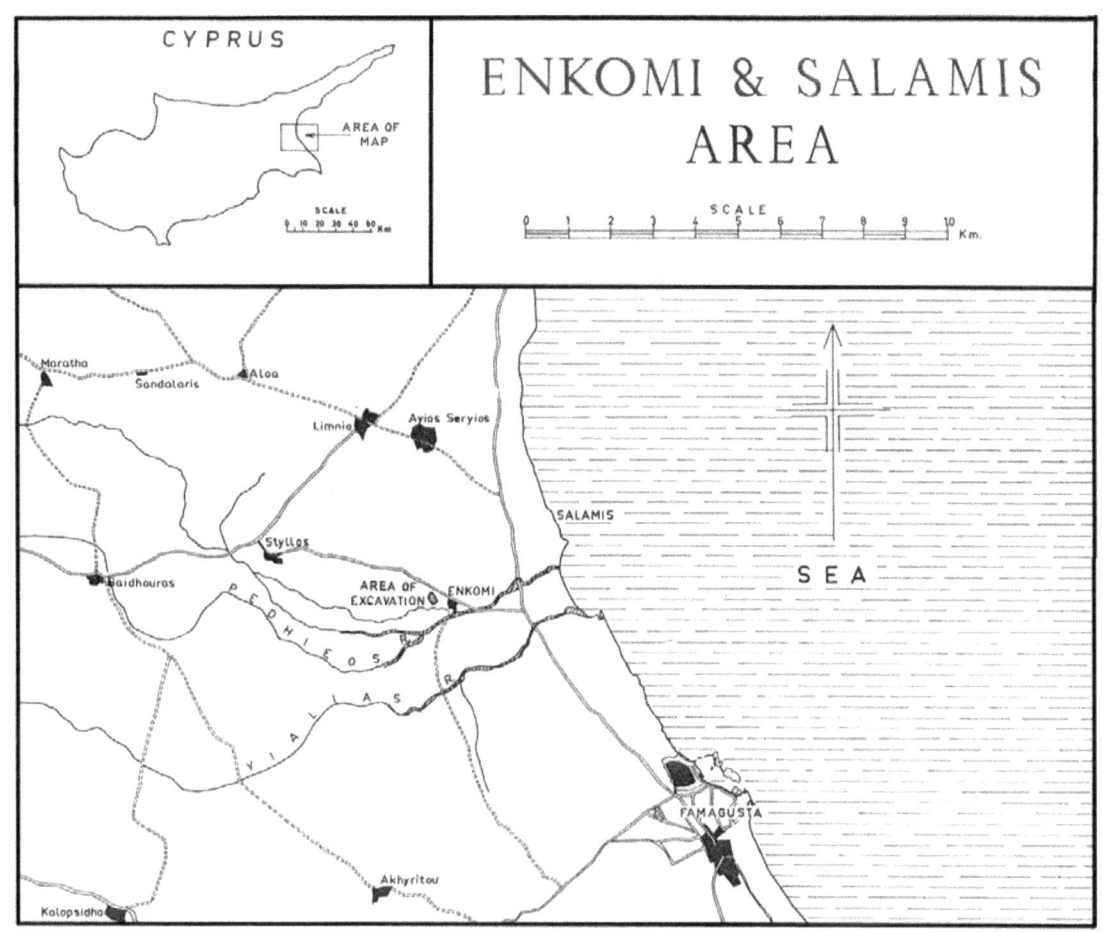

Map 11 – Enkomi general area (Dikaios 1969 plate 240)

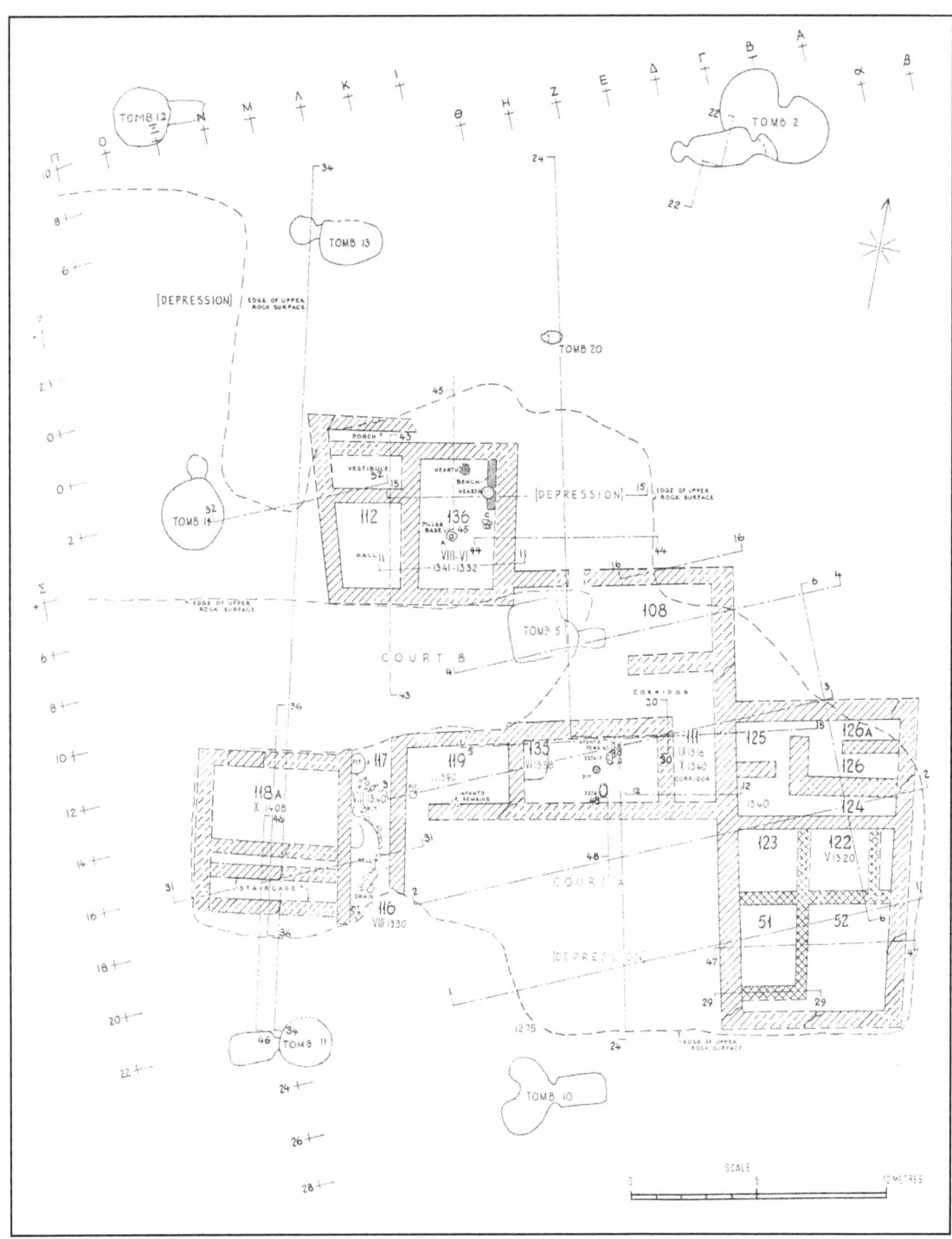

Map 12 – Enkomi excavated area (Dikaios 1969 plate 268)

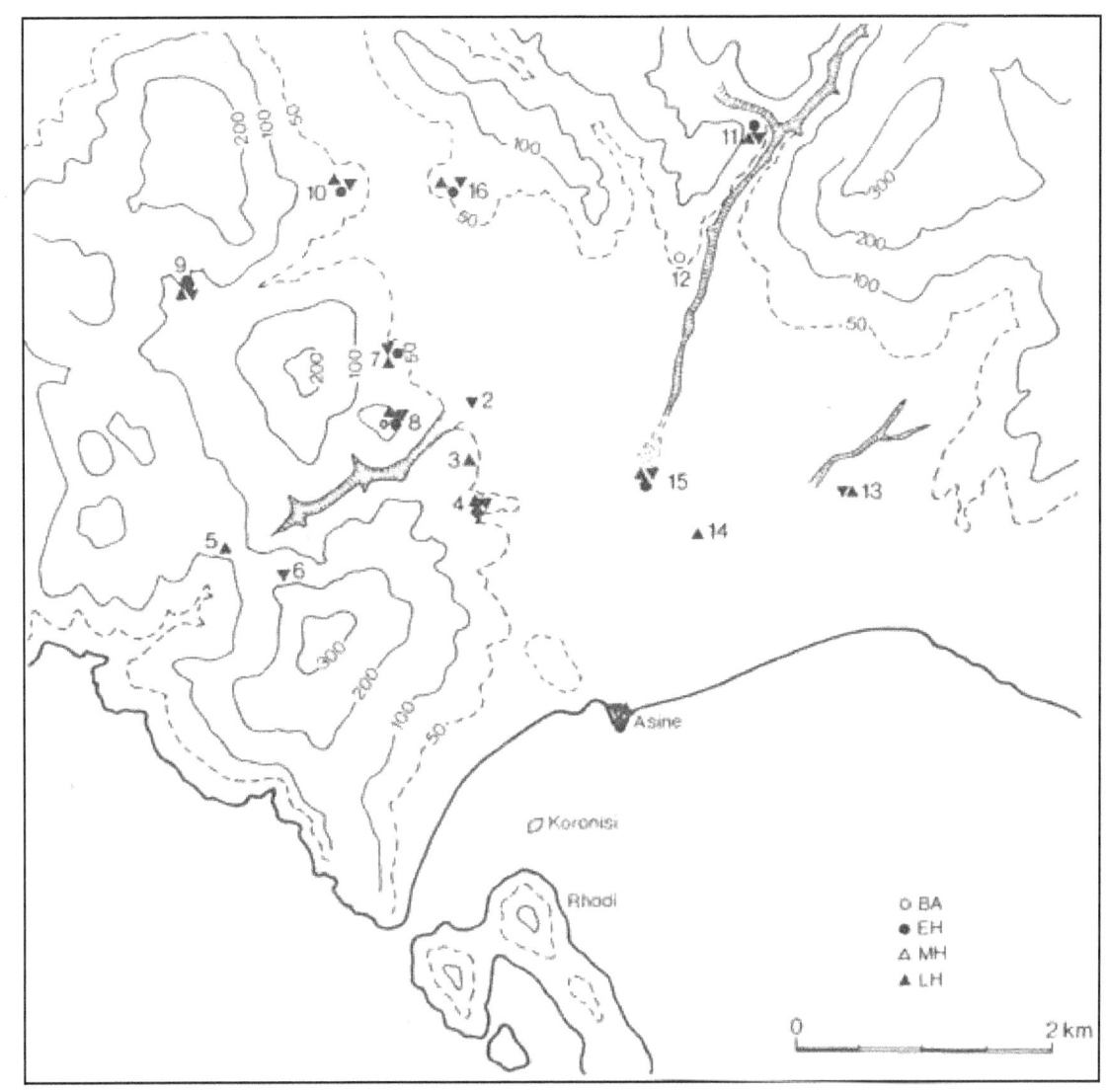

Map 13 – Asine general area (Nordquist 1987 fig 7)

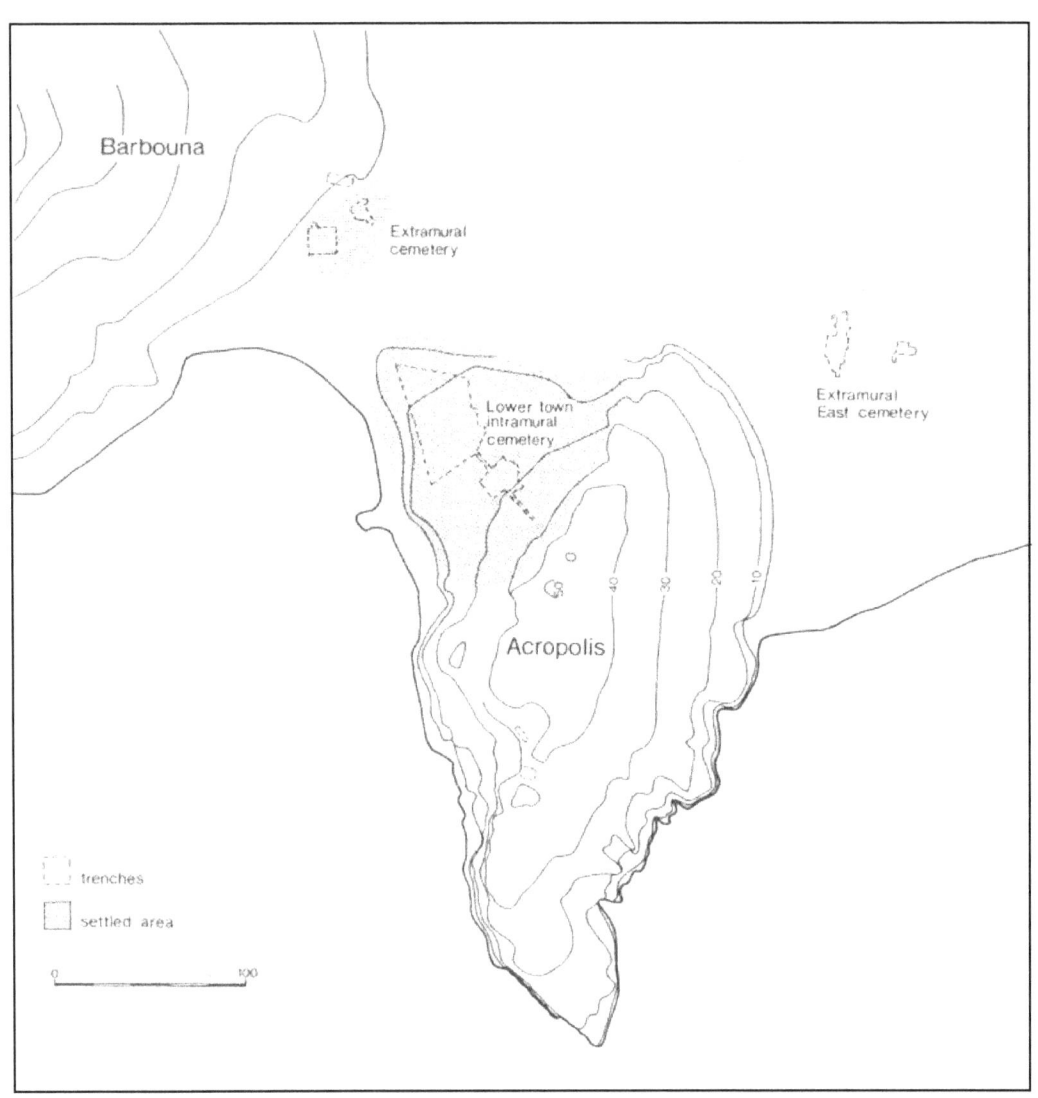

Map 14 – Asine excavated areas – Barbouna slope and Kastoraki (Nordquist 1987 fig 8)

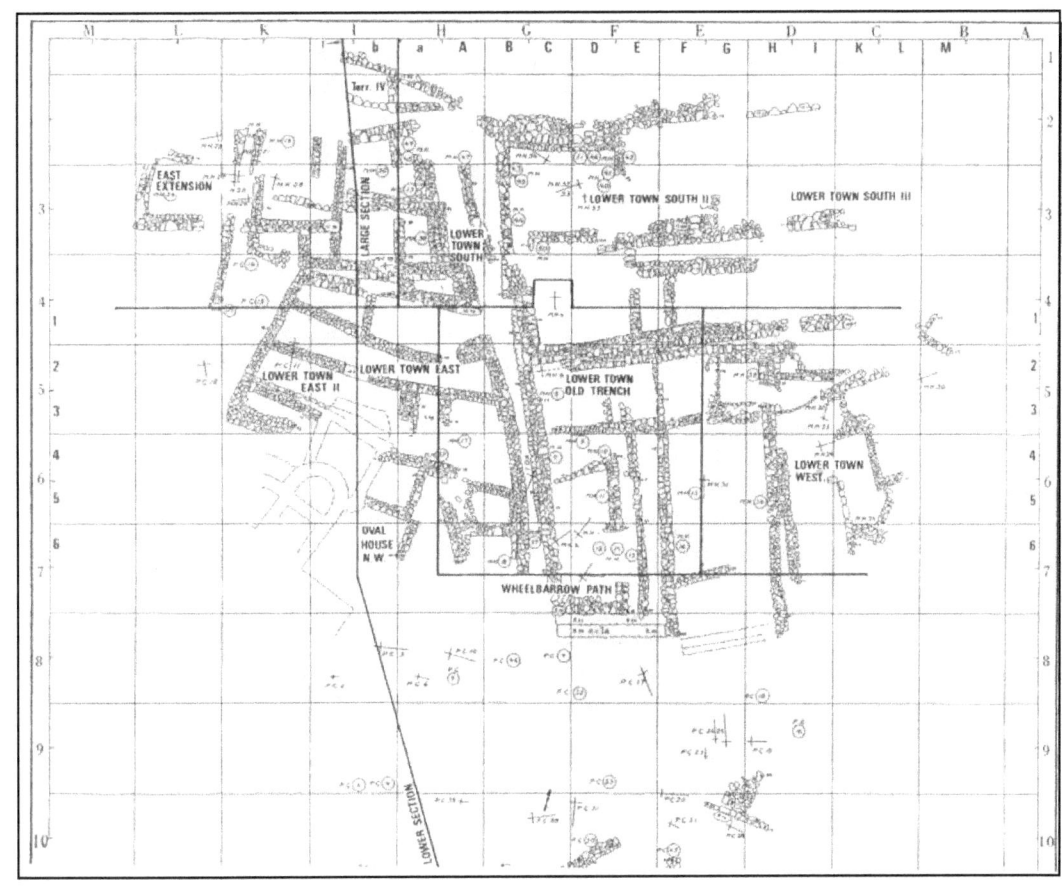

Map 15 – Asine Lower Town (Nordquist 1987 fig 5)

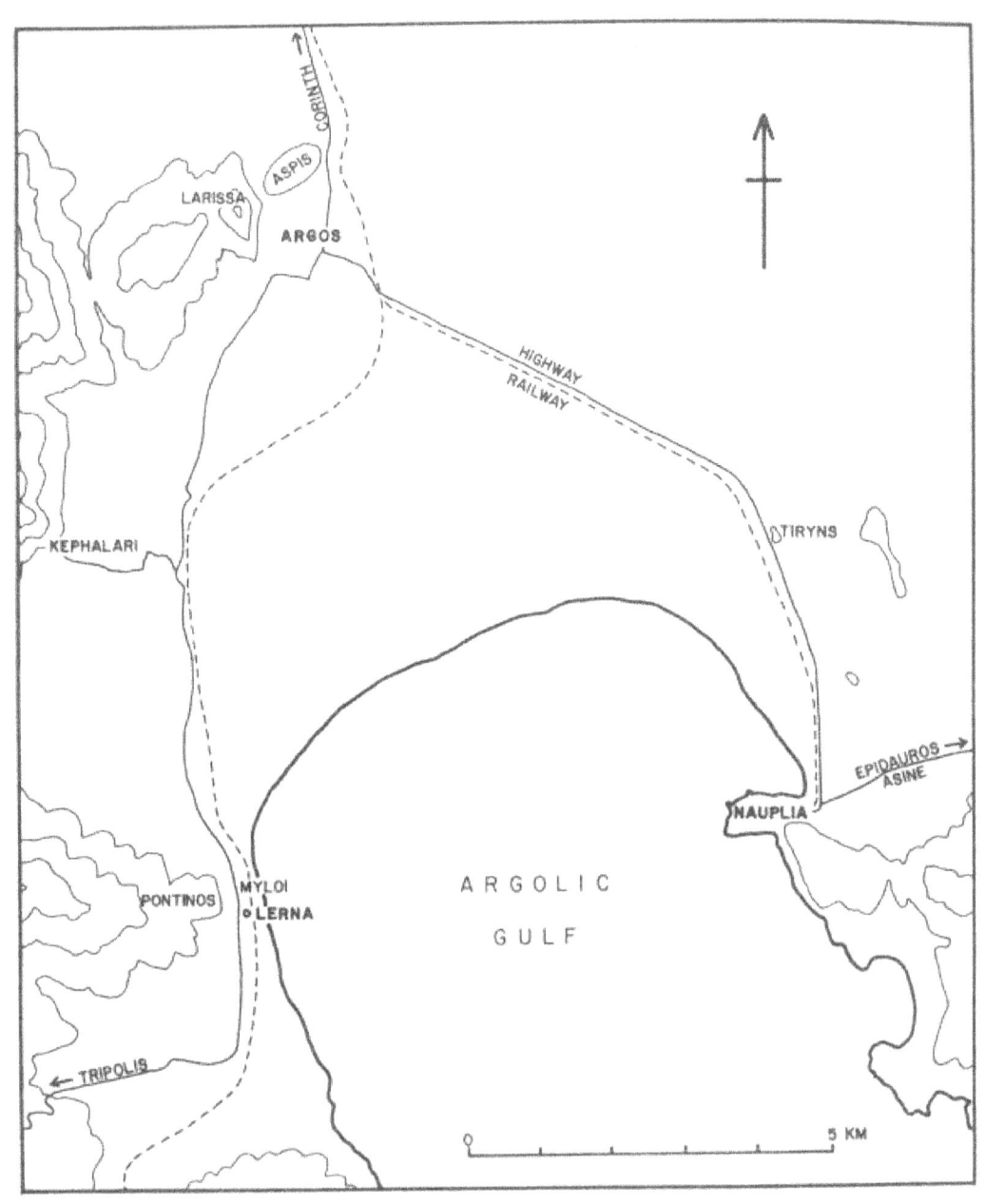

Map 16 – Lerna general area (Caskey 1997 inside cover)

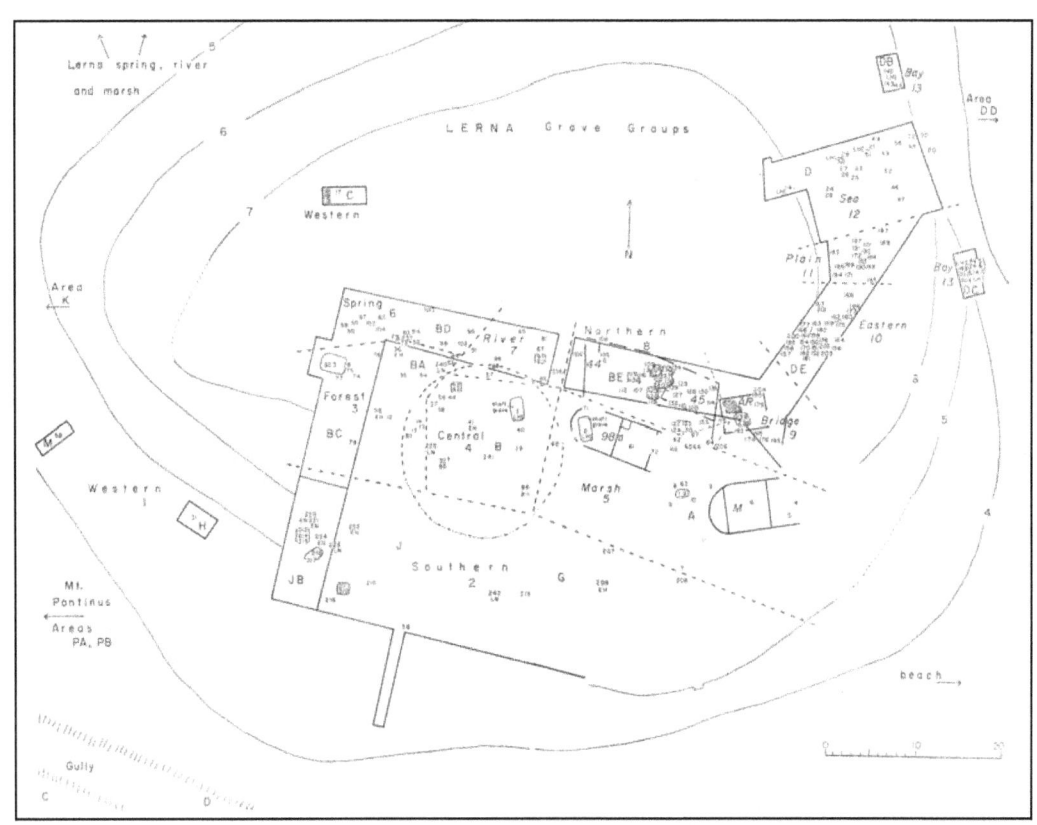

Map 17 – Lerna excavated area (Angel 1971:126-127)

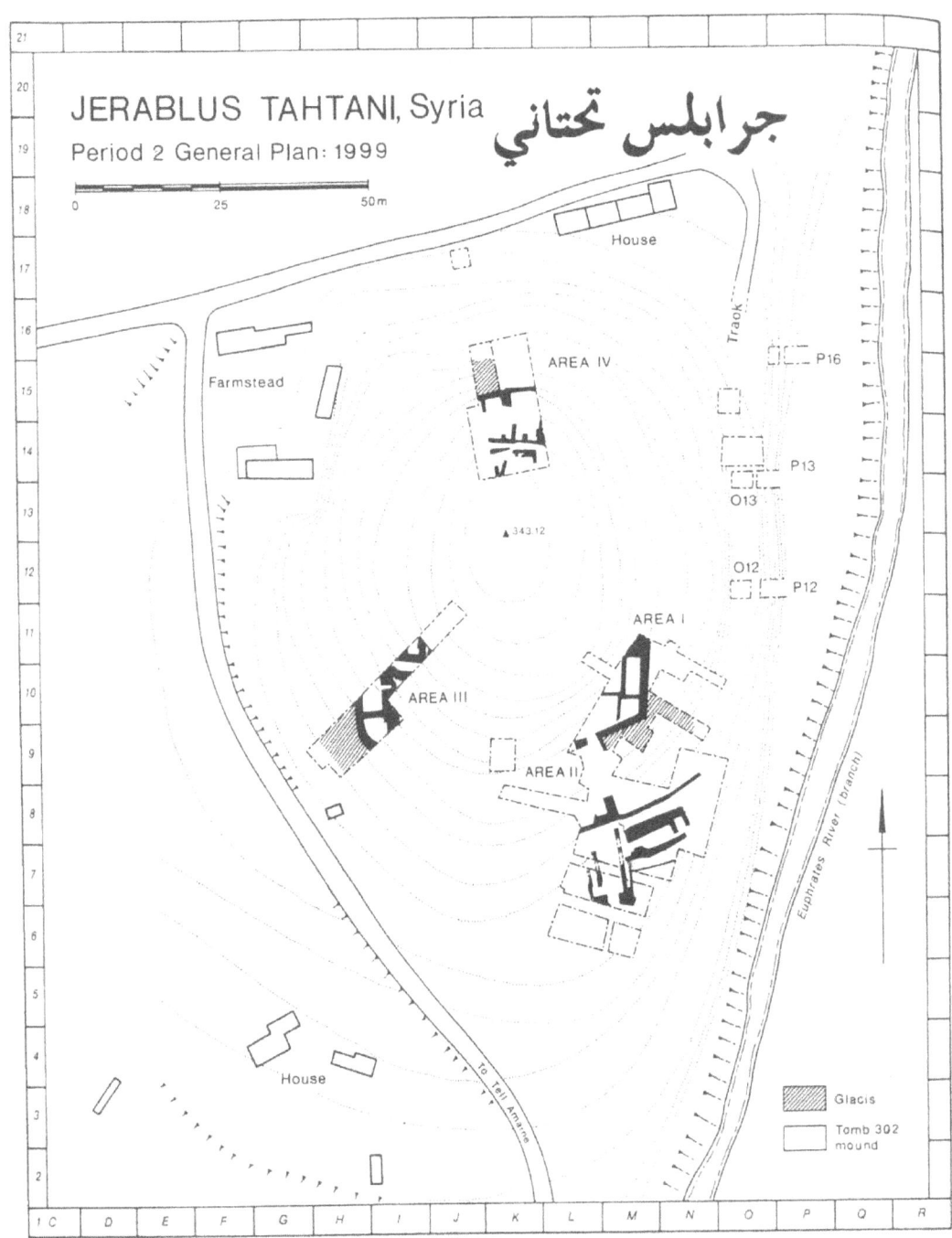

Map 18 – Jerablus-Tahtani excavated area (Peltenburg et al. 2000:54)

Lightning Source LLC
Chambersburg PA
CBHW041704290426
44108CB00027B/2848